# Contents

# Acknowledgements

The authors would like to thank the Department of Health for funding the project, while emphasising that the views expressed in the book are their own and do not necessarily represent those of the Department of Health. We would like to acknowledge the contributions of colleagues at the Thomas Coram Research Unit, Institute of Education, University of London: in particular June Statham, who directed a sister project in Wales, and at the same time made many important contributions to the English project; Julia Brannen, who provided valuable expert advice; and Pat Petrie, who carried out one of the case studies. We would also like to thank the project Advisory Committee for their guidance and support, and Peter Elfer, Susan McQuail and Gillian Pugh from the National Children's Bureau. The project has benefited from their work on services for young children, especially their evaluation of the section 19 Reviews.

Finally, we are most grateful to the local authority members and officers, to the representatives of private and voluntary sector organisations, to the community associations and to the service providers who participated in the project. We appreciate the time they so willingly gave, and for sharing their experience and knowledge with the project team. This report is based on the information, perceptions and insights they shared with us.

Thomas Coram Research Unit
Institute of Education, University of London

# *POLICY INTO PRACTICE*

# *Day Care Services for Children under Eight: an evaluation of the implementation of the Children Act*

Mano Candappa (Editor)
Julie Bull
Claire Cameron
Peter Moss
and
Charlie Owen

ISBN 0 11 321986 5

# List of abbreviations

| | |
|---|---|
| BTEC | Business and Technology Education Council |
| CQSW | Certificate of Qualification in Social Work |
| DfE | Department for Education |
| DfEE | Department for Education and Employment |
| DHSS | Department of Health and Social Security |
| DoH | Department of Health |
| DSS | Department of Social Security |
| FTE | Full-time equivalent |
| GHS | General Household Survey |
| KCN | Kids' Clubs Network |
| NCMA | National Childminding Association |
| NCH | National Children's Home |
| NEYN | National Early Years Network (formerly VOLCUF) |
| NHS | National Health Service |
| NNEB | Nursery Nursing Examination Board |
| NPDNA | National Private Day Nurseries Association |
| OPCS | Office of Population Censuses and Surveys (now the Office of National Statistics) |
| PLA | Preschool Learning Alliance (formerly Preschool Playgroups Association – PPA) |
| SSI | Social Services Inspectorate |
| TCRU | Thomas Coram Research Unit (Institute of Education, University of London) |
| TEC | Training and Enterprise Council |

# Executive Summary

This book presents the findings of the second and third stages of a four year study of the implementation of those parts of the Children Act 1989 that relate to the co-ordination, provision, regulation and support of day care services for children aged under eight years. The aim of the study has been both to monitor the implementation and to evaluate the impact of these parts of the Act, with a particular focus on day care services for children under five in England. The study was funded by the Department of Health and carried out by a research team at the Thomas Coram Research Unit (TCRU), Institute of Education, University of London. A parallel and linked study was funded by the Welsh Office and carried out in all Welsh local authorities by a member of the Thomas Coram Research Unit in Wales.

The period of the Act's introduction was one of extensive legislative and administrative change in health, welfare, and education, which has had major implications for its implementation. It coincided with a relatively new but growing interest in services for young children, and a number of policy initiatives in that area. At the same time, an increase in lone parenthood and a rapid growth in employment among women with young children has been occurring. There has also been a marked deterioration in the economic position of children and their families, with children of lone parents and from minority ethnic communities over-represented among low income households. The wider social, economic and political developments which these trends represent form the context of this study.

The first stage of the study was concerned primarily with the initial implementation of the Act and the results are reported in a previous book (Bull et al., 1994a). The present book reports on work conducted about three years after the Act's implementation and draws on the experience and views of a wider range of participants – local authority staff, providers of services and representatives of the private and voluntary sectors. The book illustrates developments and problems, and evaluates the impact of the Act in the first years of its implementation

The main findings of the second and third stages of the study reported in the book are as follows.

*Provision*

- There has been an increase in places in private day nursery and childminder provision, and in local authority nursery education provision since the Act's implementation, but not as a result of the legislation.
- Family centre provision has increased mainly through partnerships between local authorities and the voluntary sector.
- There was little change in the amount of local authority day care provision for 'children in need' (as defined under the Children Act), because planned developments were frequently offset by budget cuts.
- Sponsorship of day care places for 'children in need' in the private and voluntary sectors has increased and the range of services used has widened.
- Voluntary sector agencies reported undertaking more work with 'children in need', but few, if any, had received additional financial or advisory resources.
- Little progress has been made with planning and monitoring services for 'children in need'.
- Joint registers of children with disabilities are now in operation in most authorities.
- The Act has not led to the establishment of new day care information services, but those that exist are now better used and have a higher profile.
- Progress in making day care services more responsive to children of diverse ethnic backgrounds has been uneven and limited.

*Co-ordination*

- The Children Act has provided impetus for the development of co-ordinating structures for inter-departmental working in most authorities, many of whom had no history of working together.
- The Act has led to closer working relations between local authorities and other statutory agencies, and with the voluntary and private sectors; forums have played an important role in this process.

- The number of forums and liaison committees has increased, and they have come to play a more significant part in the development of day care services.

- There has however been little representation on co-ordinating structures of community interests such as disability and minority ethnic associations, or of users.

- The first section 19 Reviews revealed inadequacies, overlaps and gaps in services; in some cases these Reviews resulted in the establishment of co-ordinating structures.

- Despite the willingness of most local authorities to work with other agencies, achieving genuine participation by non-statutory agencies in the development of day care services has proved problematic.

*Regulation*

- The registration and inspection of day care services by independent inspection units was rather more common than by day care/under eights teams in mainstream social services departments; a few local authorities operate a split system.

- Differences exist in styles of regulation arising from different ways of organising the regulatory function and different views about the relationship between inspecting and supporting services.

- Levels of staffing for registration and inspection work differed considerably amongst local authorities.

- Inadequate staffing delayed the registration and annual inspection processes and curtailed development and support work.

- Local authorities varied considerably in their approach to assessing whether a potential provider was a 'fit person' and to issues of ethnic diversity.

- Following Circular LAC (93)1 and the case of the Sutton childminder, there was a climate of uncertainty about the role and status of regulation in maintaining standards and promoting quality.

- The power to cancel or refuse registration has not been used widely; authorities have mostly worked with service providers over a period of time or counselled them out of the registration process where necessary.

- Service providers seem to have adjusted to the new regulatory regime over the period of implementation, with widespread acceptance for the principle of regulation; inspection has largely been experienced as positive and most providers have regarded the standards set by their local authority as 'about right'.
- There was little evidence that the implementation of the Children Act, in particular the new regulatory regime, affected growth in provision.
- Service providers' responses to the new regulatory regime have varied between local authorities; generally, day nurseries have been more critical than other providers.

*Support*

- Offering advice and providing training has played a secondary role to regulation.
- None of the local authorities in the sample had a formula for determining an appropriate level of staffing for supporting day care providers.
- On the whole, workloads have been too large to offer adequate support, even in local authorities where there are 'dedicated' support workers.
- Most local authorities have provided some funding to voluntary organisations, which then provided various forms of support to service providers, but the amounts of funding were usually small.
- Most service providers felt there was someone they could contact for advice and support, usually local authority staff, and had made regular contact which they generally found helpful; day nurseries were more critical than other providers.
- Most service providers wanted more training but many have had difficulty in finding or attending training courses, in particular due to difficulties with timing, cover to release staff, costs, transport and lack of childcare.
- Service providers who have received extra help when taking 'children in need' generally appreciated this support; but a substantial proportion have not received additional help and would have liked some.

- Overall the Children Act was seen as neutral or mildly positive in its effect on levels of support for service providers.

*Parents*

- The Children Act required local authorities to consult with parents and most – if not all – had done so.

- Some authorities had adopted innovative strategies for contacting parents and these deserve to be more widely disseminated and emulated.

- Few local authorities had conducted a formal survey of parents, but those that had often failed to obtain representative samples.

- Some guidance on the conduct of surveys would be beneficial, as would co-ordination between surveys, including the inclusion of some common questions.

- Views expressed by parents agreed with what has been found by national sample surveys: parents want more nursery education, more day nurseries, longer hours (especially for playgroups) and less expensive day care.

*Conclusions*

- Overall, the Children Act has produced a number of worthwhile but modest improvements in day care services for children under eight.

- There are a number of issues which cut across findings for the specific themes of provision, co-ordination, regulation and support, including: resource constraints; the need to give more attention to the conditions required to meet the high expectations placed on the private and voluntary sectors; inadequacy of information; the different points that local authorities started from in their implementation of the Children Act; and the marginalisation and division of services for young children.

- More attention needs to be given to improving the range and quality of information at local and national levels to support the development of services and strengthen the effectiveness of the Act. This requires regular information collected from and about families (demand, need and use of services) and services themselves.

- After five years of operation, it is a good time to reflect on the working of the Act as it applies to day care services. This process of reflection could consider the feasibility of working within the existing structure of the Act and associated Guidance, developing this structure in the light of experience. A second approach could involve a more general review of policy and services for children aged under eight years, that would consider *inter alia* the most appropriate legal framework for these services.

CHAPTER

# 1 Introduction

**Julie Bull and Peter Moss**

Since the implementation of the 1989 Children Act in 1991, a research team at the Thomas Coram Research Unit, Institute of Education, University of London, has been studying the consequences of the Act for day care services for children aged under eight years. This book is the latest in a series of publications from the study, and focuses on the Children Act three years after implementation. Before saying more about the study and the scope of the book, we begin this introductory chapter by looking at the Act and the context in which it has been implemented.

## The Children Act

*Duties, powers and principles*

The Children Act, a major piece of legislation consolidating almost all previous private and public law relating to children, was implemented in 1991 following an unusually lengthy process of consultation. The greater part of the Act concerns private law and the role of social work and the courts in relation to specific groups of children, including what the Act refers to as 'children in need', a group covering children with disabilities as well as children with actual or potential problems of health or development. Part III of the Act not only introduces and broadly defines the concept of 'children in need', but places a duty on local authorities to provide 'family support services' for these children and their families. Day care services (defined as day nurseries, playgroups, childminders and out-of school services for children aged 5–7 years) are specifically recognised in this part of the Act as 'family support services'.

While the larger part of the Act's treatment of day care services relates to this welfare role for children 'in need', there are also important duties relating to day care services in general use. In particular, the Act places a duty on local authorities to regulate services in the private and voluntary sectors and a further duty to undertake a triennial Review of day care services. The main duties and powers relating to day care services within the new legal framework are summarised below (see Box 1.1).

In constituting a statement of policy on *services for young children* (a term we use to cover the full range of day care services for children aged under eight and of education services for children under five), the Act itself needs to be considered together with two subsequent documents: Volume Two of the Children Act Guidance and Regulations (hereafter referred to as 'Guidance') (DoH, 1991) and Circular LAC (93)1 issued by the Department of Health in January 1993, both of which were intended to add further clarification and guidance for local authorities in interpreting the Act. Guidance focuses in particular on clarifying the process of registration and inspection.

**Box 1.1**

**Day care services: duties placed on local authorities by the Children Act**

- A general duty to provide day care services for children who are in need and their families, to publicise the services available to children in need, and to have regard to the different racial groups to which children in need belong (Part III sections.17 and 18).
- A general duty to provide such family centres as [local authorities] consider appropriate to children within their area (Schedule 2).
- A duty to regulate most private and voluntary day care services (Part X).
- A joint duty for education and social services departments to conduct a Review of day care services for children aged under eight at least once every three years (section 19).

**Day care services: powers given to local authorities by the Children Act**

- A power to provide day care for children not in need (section 18).
- A power to provide support for day care providers (such as training, guidance and counselling (section 18).

Circular LAC (93)1 also focuses on clarifying the regulatory role. While asserting that the child's welfare 'is the paramount consideration' in regulation, the Circular also expects local authorities to set standards in terms of their impact on the supply of services – 'local authorities should operate their registration systems in a constructive and flexible way to ensure standards and encourage expansion of day care facilities' (para. 12). Local authorities should not be setting standards that are 'unrealistically high to the point where they inhibit expansion'.

There are two points about the Act in relation to these duties and powers which are important in assessing its overall significance for services for young children. They have been discussed at length elsewhere (Cameron and Moss, 1995; Bull et al., 1996) but are reviewed briefly here. The first point is that educational services for children aged under five (nursery classes and schools and reception classes for four year-olds) remain outside the framework of the Children Act. They are not included in the Review duty which relates primarily to day care services, although the Review is supposed to 'take account of nursery and primary education facilities' (DoH, 1991: para. 9.2); nor are they subject to the same regulatory regime. The Act therefore retains both the practical and conceptual divide between day care and education that has historically underpinned services for young children in the UK and focuses specifically on day care.

Secondly, there are no general legal or other principles which apply across all parts of the Act and the application of all powers and duties. For example, the principle that the welfare of the child should be a paramount consideration applies only to Section 1 of the Act in relation to the work of the courts. It does not apply generally to all parts of the Act, for example to the regulatory function for general day care services. The specificity of the paramountcy principle was confirmed in a Court of Appeal ruling (cf. *Re M (a Minor)*, Court of Appeal, 10 November 1994), where Lady Justice Butler Sloss concluded that 'the general duty of a local authority to safeguard and promote the child's welfare [under Part 3 of the Act] is not the same as that imposed upon the court in s.1 placing welfare as the paramount consideration'.

Although Guidance refers to this paramountcy principle, it does so as one of several principles that 'should inform good practice in day care, education and related services' (ibid.: para. 6.2), a statement of intent that falls far short of requiring local authorities to apply the principle in the performance of their regulatory duty. Similarly, Circular LAC (93)1, as already noted, first says that children's welfare should be 'the paramount consideration' in registration. Yet, it immediately qualifies this statement by implying that other considerations, which could well be in conflict, in particular ensuring a supply of services, should be taken account of in the operation of registration.

*Expectations and limitations*

At the time of the presentation of the then Children Bill to the House of Lords, the new legislation was described by the Lord Chancellor as 'the most comprehensive and far-reaching reform of child care law which has come before Parliament in living memory'. The provisions which relate to day care form a relatively small part of this overall reform and were not the outcome of the extensive preceding review and debate which informed other sections of the legislation (Cameron and Moss, 1995). Expectations of what the Act could deliver for services for young children, however, were high. The Act was universally welcomed in day care circles as representing a more coherent framework for the provision of day care services, in particular for the strategic approach signalled by the introduction of the three yearly Review duty, for the duty to provide publicly funded day care for children 'in need', for the unprecedented attention it gave to children's ethnic, cultural and linguistic diversity, as well as for the more rigorous standards introduced by the new modernised registration system. Generally, many hoped that the Act would help to bring day care services into greater prominence from the historically marginalised position they have occupied in most social services departments.

While innovatory in some important details, closer analysis of the Children Act's assumptions and objectives for day care services shows them to be conservative in essence, introducing a note of caution into expectations of what the Act might achieve. In essence, the Act consolidates existing and long-standing policy on day care. In terms of public responsibility for the provision of day care, the Act refines and reinforces a limited welfare role, placing it within the broader concept of 'children in need'. For the great majority of children, the provision of day care continues to be deemed a private matter, for which parents are entirely responsible. Access to day care services, therefore, continues to depend on parental purchasing power within a largely unsubsidised private market of provision; Guidance makes it clear that the power given to local authorities to provide day care for children not 'in need' is not expected to be widely exercised (cf. DoH, 1991, para.4.8). The Act and Guidance assume the validity of a continuing distinction between day care and education for young children, and the retention of a structural divide of services for young children between the welfare and education systems; as for many years, greater co-ordination between these two systems is the model that is assumed and encouraged. In reforming the regulatio. services, the Act builds on a long-standing role for local authorities in reg istering and inspecting services for young children.

The Act and Guidance can therefore be seen as measures to consolidate and improve, rather than reform, policy. As a consequence, the Act and Guidance do not address important, long-standing and much debated questions about services for young children. The question of the cost and distribution of services, which are currently variable and uneven, is not tackled. While the Act and Guidance pay considerable attention to ethnic, linguistic and cultural diversity, they ignore socio-economic diversity, an important omission in a period of increasing child poverty and financial inequality between families and when the main strategy for provision relies on parents buying services in a private market. At the same time as confirming this strategy for provision, the Act and Guidance introduce an enhanced model of public regulation of that private market, and in so doing increase existing tension between standards, supply and access. Differences in standards and principles of access between day care and education services, reflecting large cultural differences between the welfare and education systems, are documented in Guidance, but not considered in the context of their implications for co-ordination. The following chapters explore some of the tensions arising from these unresolved issues, which in some ways have been made more acute by the implementation of the Act.

## The Context

*The climate of implementation*

The Children Act has been introduced in a climate of extensive legislative and administrative change which has had major implications for its implementation. The NHS and Community Care Act 1990 and the Criminal Justice Act 1991 were implemented almost concurrently with the Children Act by social services departments. Education departments have faced a series of major reforms since the early 1980s, which in many respects have undermined co-ordination of services for young children between social services and education, in particular following from local management of schools (Pugh, 1992). Boundary changes to local authorities will have major implications for the planning and co-ordination of services for young children.

There is a growing interest in services providing day care and education for children aged under five and providing care and recreation for school-age children, among a widening range of public bodies. This has been reflected in a number of recent policy initiatives, which have coincided with the implementation of the Children Act and indicate the growing importance attached by Government to these services. For example, the then Employment Department announced an Out of School Childcare Initiative in 1992, and at a local level, TECs have become involved with the Out of School Childcare Initiative and also with day care services for younger children. In 1994, a subsidy for the day care costs of some low income benefit claimants (the childcare disregard) was introduced by the Department of Social Security. Most recently, a growing 'consensus that education provision for under-fives is beneficial' (Audit Commission, 1996: 7), reflected in two major reports (National Commission on Education, 1993; Ball, C., 1994), has found expression in a Government commitment to offer a 'pre-school place' for all 4 year olds, and to deliver this through a voucher scheme. This aims to enable parents to purchase five half-day sessions in any approved form of provision (in the public, voluntary or private sector) of their choice. The scheme, which has been developed by the DfEE, began its first stage of implementation in April 1996, with general implementation planned for a year later. The voucher scheme also includes a new 'light touch' inspection regime for those institutions wishing to participate in the scheme.

These recent initiatives will increase access to services. But a feature of them, which again relates to the effectiveness of the strategy of co-ordination that underpins policy in the area of services for young children, is that they have all (including the Children Act) originated from different government departments. Although there are some mechanisms for inter-departmental co-ordination (i.e. Cabinet committees, a Ministerial Group on Under Eights), it is not clear whether or how these mechanisms have been brought to bear on recent policy initiatives, and there is no shared inter-departmental policy on services for young children to underpin the coordination of individual departmental initiatives. Each initiative has emerged independently in response to different departmental agendas, rather than as a concerted contribution to the development of a common policy on services for young children.

Social and economic changes have also crucially affected the context in which the Children Act, as part of other policy initiatives, has been implemented. Recent decades have witnessed important and now well documented trends in patterns of family life that have produced increasing diversity in household circumstances and structure, and expose children and parents to increasing change and transition in all aspects of their lives. Three trends are particularly important and relevant to the subject of this book.

First, there has been a rapid increase in lone parenthood. The proportion of families headed by a lone parent rose from 8 per cent in 1971 to 22 per cent in 1993, mainly due to an increase in lone mother families. The proportion of lone mothers increased gradually until 1987, since when it has grown rapidly (OPCS, 1995, fig 2E; Central Statistical Office, 1995).

Second, there has been rapid growth of employment among women with young children, especially since the mid-1980s. Between 1985 and 1994, for example, the employment rate among mothers of children aged under five increased from 30 per cent to 46 per cent; with a further 6 per cent looking for work, a majority of women with young children are now economically active (GHS, 1995). This increase in employment however has not been uniform: employment has grown fastest among women who are highly qualified, white and living with an employed partner; it has grown least or declined among lone mothers, Afro-Caribbean mothers, women with lower levels of qualification and women with partners who are unemployed. At a household level, there are more two-earner families but also more no-earner households – producing the phenomenon of more 'work rich' and more 'work poor' families (Harrop and Moss, 1994; Brannen et al., 1994).

Moreover, although most employed women with a child aged under five have part-time jobs, the proportion with full-time jobs has begun to increase. Between 1985 and 1994, full-time employment grew at twice the rate of part-time employment. There has also been a rapid increase in the proportion of women resuming work after maternity leave, pointing to increasing parental employment in families with very young children (under 2 years) (McRae, 1991).

But it is not just the amount and distribution of employment that is changing; it is the nature of employment itself. New technology and growing competition, deregulation and increasing flexibility in the labour market may open up new opportunities for some workers and their families. But they may also mean increased insecurity and intensification of work for many others, producing what has been described by Hutton (1995) as a 30/30/40 society – the first 30 per cent being the unemployed and economically inactive, the second 30 per cent being people whose jobs are insecure, poorly protected and carry few benefits, while the remaining 40 per cent are relatively privileged workers in relatively secure jobs. Hutton relates this economic analysis to the condition of families with children: 'the fact that more than half the people in Britain who are eligible to work are living either on poverty incomes or in conditions of permanent stress and insecurity...makes it harder and harder for men and women in these circumstances to hold their marriages together let alone parent their children adequately' (ibid.: 109).

Third, and related closely to the previous two trends, there has been a deterioration in the economic position of children and their families. In a context of growing variation in income, the proportion of children living in families whose income is below half the national average (one definition of poverty) has grown three-fold to stand now at 1 in 3[1]. The children of lone parents and of minority ethnic groups are over-represented among low income households (Kumar, 1993); for example, in 1993 67 per cent of lone mother households had a gross weekly income below £150 compared to just 12 per cent of couple households (OPCS, 1995, table 2.30).

The overall picture therefore is one of growing diversity in the situation of families, with some enjoying increasing opportunities and income, while the position of others is increasingly precarious and insecure – and all within a context of increasing social and economic change. These trends have important consequences for the needs of children and their families in relation to services for young children, for the demands being made of these services and for the ability of families to access them. They raise questions about what types of services are needed to respond to increasing diversity and change in the circumstances of young children and their families – and about the most appropriate legal framework for these services.

## Day Care Services

*Current day care provision*

Day care provision encompasses a wide range of services, from family centres to childminders, and from day nurseries to playgroups; there is great diversity both within and between these different types of service. An earlier book (Bull et al., 1994a) detailed the position of day care services at the time of the Children Act's implementation and discussed the shortcomings of statistical sources at some length. Only a brief update therefore is provided here.

In 1994, there were 914,000 places at day nurseries, playgroups and childminders in England as recorded in official statistics (see Table 1.1). This

1. For more information on the economic situation of children, families and the general population, see: Department of Social Security (DSS), 1993; Kumar, 1993; Commission on Social Justice, 1994; Jenkins, 1994; Goodman and Wells, 1994; Central Statistical Office, 1995.

does not provide a complete picture of day care provision for children under five years. It *excludes* family centres, a growing area of provision by both local authorities and voluntary organisations. Official statistics tell us that in 1994 there were 380 family centres provided by local authorities taking children under five, but there is no information on the number of places provided in these centres. However, it does *include* places at childminders for both children under five, and between five and eight, but there is no way of knowing how in practice these places divide between the two age groups.

Although it is not possible, for these reasons, to make a precise assessment of the number of day care places for children under five, in broad terms there are *places* equivalent to around 25–30 per cent of the age group, although the nature of these places varies considerably. The 1990 OPCS survey reported that 35 per cent of *children* under five were attending registered childminders, playgroups and day nurseries, reflecting the fact that some places, especially in playgroups, are used by more than one child on a part-time basis (Meltzer, 1994, table 4.1).

Large numbers of children are also cared for in informal arrangements, for example with relatives or friends (Brannen et al., 1994). In addition, there are day care services providing out-of-school care for children aged 5-8 years, some provided by childminders, others in 'out-of-school clubs' and other centres. The 1994 DoH returns show that there were approximately 30,000 places for 5-8 year olds in 'out of school clubs', 30 per cent provided by local authorities, the rest by private providers, equivalent to about 1.5 per cent of the age group.

*Recent trends*

Table 1.1 also shows trends in day care provision for children aged under five from 1985 to 1994, that is both before and after the implementation of the Children Act. There is a decrease in local authority run provision, due mainly to a substantial fall in day nursery provision since 1991. Most day care provision, however (over 95 per cent), is provided by voluntary organisations or privately, and this independent sector has been growing since 1985. Playgroups form the largest group within the independent sector, but there has been little change in levels of provision since 1985, and indeed some decline in places since 1991. The DoH (1995a) suggests that this decline may owe something to the Children Act, but static provision may also be due to playgroups having reached a ceiling of demand, which is gradually lowering due to increased education provision for children under five. McQuail and Pugh (1995: 3) confirm the likely impact of education services on playgroups, concluding that a fall in playgroup provision 'is a consequence of the pressure for earlier admissions to schools, combined with the competitive pressures of local management of schools'.

**Table 1.1: Places in main types of day care provision for children under five (1994) and changes in provision (1985–1994): England**

| *Type of provision* | *Number. of places and places per 100 children 0-5 years* | | *Change in number of places: 85–88* | *88–91* | *91–94* |
|---|---|---|---|---|---|
| *Local authority run provision* | *26,000* | *[0.8%]* | *+1%* | *–7%* | *–12%* |
| Day nurseries | 22,300 | [0.7%] | | | |
| Childminders | 2,100 | * | | | |
| Playgroups | 1,600 | * | | | |
| *Places paid for by local authorities* | *21,400* | *[0.7%]* | *+34%* | *+7%* | *+4%* |
| *Private providers* | *890,400* | *[27.4%]* | *+9%* | *+22%* | *+21%* |
| Day nurseries | 125,300 | [3.9%] | +44% | +120% | +59% |
| Childminders | 355,400 | [11.0%] | +29% | +43% | +54% |
| Playgroups | 409,700 | [12,6%] | –* | +5% | –4% |

* less than 0.5%

Source: DoH, 1995a, table 1

The main areas of growth among private providers have therefore been private day nurseries and childminders. The most rapid rate of growth for day nurseries was between 1988 and 1991, and the rate has fallen somewhat since 1991. However, this probably has little to do with any inhibiting effects of the Children Act. Growth in private day nurseries accelerated dramatically in the mid-1980s, from a low base and after a long period when there was little change. This 'take off' was most likely due to the rapid increase in employment rates among women with young children which occurred from the mid-1980s onwards, and which we have already noted was particularly strong for full-time employment among higher educated women, who are the main users of private day nurseries. The very rapid *growth rate* for 1988–91 was therefore a consequence of the previously low levels of private day nursery provision: in fact, in terms of *new places* opened each year, the post-1991 period showed faster growth (15,636 extra places per year between 1991 and 1994) than the 1988–91 period (13,613 extra places per year).

Growth in childminding also increased after 1988 and, unlike day nurseries, the growth rate was even faster after 1991. However, this post-1991 change is difficult to interpret. An accurate picture of trends in childminding provision is hampered by the fact that some childminders registered before the Act may have been doing little or no minding in practice; any reduction in numbers due to the Act resulted mainly or wholly from 'weeding out' these essentially inactive childminders, rather then removing active but inadequate providers. In effect, therefore, a reduction in registered childminders may not have led to a fall in the effective supply of provision. However, these changes resulting from the process of implementing the Children Act should have stabilised by 1993; the significant increase that occurred between 1993 and 1994 in both the number of childminders registered (+11 per cent) and the number of registered places (+20 per cent) suggests therefore that the growth observed before 1991 is continuing.

Overall, it is impossible to get an accurate picture of trends in *private* day care services. However, it can be concluded that there has been a substantial increase among some types of providers in the private sector, and there seems little evidence that the implementation of the Children Act affected real growth in provision (an issue discussed further in chapter 5). It is more likely that the main factor influencing growth has been changes in the extent and nature of maternal employment and, in the case of playgroups, growth in the availability of school-based services. Trends in *publicly funded* day care provision, and any impact of the Children Act on public provision, is equally difficult to assess, but there is little evidence of a substantial increase from a historically low level of provision.

*The main features of day care services*

Private day care services for young children are in many ways different to other private services for which the welfare system has some responsibility, for example residential services for disabled or elderly people. There are a large number of them, some 118,500 childminders, playgroups, private day nurseries and out-of-school clubs. Mostly, they consist of numerous individual carers working from home, and small, part-time non-profit centres. While the number of full-time, for-profit businesses (private day nurseries) is growing, they account for less than 5 per cent of all the private day care services; even these centres are relatively small-scale, with an average of 28 places per registered day nursery.

In 1993, there were 5,200 staff employed in local authority run nurseries and playgroups (DoH, 1995a, table 9). Otherwise, there is little information about this workforce, although some features are apparent. First, levels of training are in general low: the basic NNEB training is at a two-year post-16 level, but most day care workers either have training at a lower level than the NNEB or none at all. Second, staff are overwhelmingly female: in a recent survey of service providers conducted by Thomas Coram Research Unit (Moss et al., 1995; further information about the survey is given later in this chapter), 99 per cent of childminders were female, and only 14 per cent of nurseries and 8 per cent of playgroups had any male staff. According to the 1991 Census, the occupational group 'child care and related occupations' was the most gender segregated occupation with over 98 per cent of workers female. Third, services are more likely to have minority ethnic children than to have minority ethnic staff; in the service providers survey, playgroups and nurseries were twice as likely to have minority ethnic children as to have minority ethnic staff. Fourth, pay and employment conditions are generally poor, especially in the private sector (Moss and Penn, 1996).

Although the day care services on offer are diverse and cover a range of functions, in practice the choice actually available to a parent is less than might seem apparent, for a number of reasons:

- **The narrow remit of services**: rather than being multi-functional in approach, most day care services are mainly in the business of performing one function, be it care, education or support. For example private day nurseries are intended mainly to provide care for children of employed parents, while local authority day nurseries are for children 'in need' rather than children of employed parents. Services vary in their opening hours and the age group of children they take; the service providers survey showed that most (but not all) childminders and private nurseries took children under two, but very few playgroups did; playgroups were open for short hours (less than 15 hours a week on average, in school terms only), a third of childminders described themselves as part-time and day nurseries were generally open throughout the year and, on average, for 48 hours a week.
- **Cost**: the great majority of places in day care services are unsubsidised and parents must therefore be able and willing to pay for a

place. Average fees reported in the service providers survey were similar for nurseries and childminders (around £1.70 per hour), but half this level for playgroups. However, there will be considerable variations between individual services, reflecting location (fees being higher in London), the age of child (fees being higher for very young children) and standards (for example, services with better qualified staff and better physical environments are likely to cost more). In a 1994 survey of childminders, NCMA found an average hourly rate of £1.60 (very similar to the service providers survey average), but with variations from £1.10 to £4 an hour. While the child care disregard introduced in 1994 was intended to introduce an element of subsidy for some low income families using private services, so far it has had a limited impact. At the end of July 1995, only 19,000 lone parents were claiming the disregard, which was far below official projections (Mr Andrew Mitchell, Written Parliamentary answer, 11 December 1995).

- **Distribution:** the DoH's own statistics show very clearly a wide variation in provision of all types of day care services between local authorities (DoH, 1995a, tables E and I). A recent report notes 'a wide variation in children's access to services, an issue which should be of concern to local authorities that wish to improve under-fives' participation in education' (Audit Commission, 1996: 14).

These features of day care providers contribute an important part of the context within which the potential and actual impact of the Children Act must be considered. We will return to their significance in later chapters. We also return in the final chapter to consider the need for improved statistics to provide a proper information base for monitoring day care services.

*Local authorities and services for young children*

The diverse and fragmented nature of the provision of services for young children is also dominated by great variation between local authorities. Such variations reflect different political priorities and professional values which are in turn reflected in local authorities' resourcing, organisation, management and co-ordination of services for young children. Against a backdrop of overall low levels of public funding for day care, some authorities have achieved relatively high levels of publicly-funded provision and have attempted to provide services to a wide range of children, while others have maintained a relatively narrow role for public day care as part of child protection services. In terms of co-ordination, within local authorities themselves there are usually two or sometimes three departments involved in the provision of services for young children, each operating within different legislative contexts but also each having their own different underpinning philosophies and language reflecting an underlying emphasis on either care, education or play (Penn and Riley, 1992).

In the late 1980s, however, a number of authorities began to review this traditional departmental split in the organisation of services for young children and to move towards a more integrated structure combining both care and education services within a single department. These were usually authorities with a high level of political commitment to services for young children, high levels of publicly funded welfare and education provision and a belief in a general right of access to services. At the time of the Children Act's implementation, some authorities had already effected the transition to an integrated structure, and more have followed since, although such authorities are in the minority and the dominant model remains the 'traditional' one, of services provided by separate departments. Within this majority model however, can be found widely different emphases in the balance between direct and indirect provision of services, the scope and degree of inter-departmental working and the overall policy approach to services for young children (McQuail and Pugh, 1995).

The importance of this variance is that the Children Act was received within very different local contexts. It had a different significance for different authorities and was interpreted around existing and very different patterns of provision, priorities for access to services, and departmental boundaries and culture. For example, an authority which had a historical commitment to provide services along universalist, non-stigmatising lines would be more likely to interpret the definition of 'in need' in a broad or inclusive way than an authority which had a child protection focus to the provision of day care services. Equally, an authority with an integrated service would approach the co-ordination function differently from one with separate departments. Although these are two obvious examples, they illustrate the extent to which local authorities had different starting points from which to take forward the Children Act, which crucially affects how much change may have come about as a consequence of its implementation and the overall significance of the Act in the long-term development of policy and services.

## The project

*Design and Methods*

The research findings presented in this volume come from a project undertaken by the Thomas Coram Research Unit for the Department of Health between 1992 and 1995. The aim of the project was both to monitor the implementation and to evaluate the impact of the parts of the Act which affect day care services. The focus of the project was day care services for children under five in England. A separate but linked study, funded by the Welsh Office, took place at the same time throughout Wales, the findings of which are reported separately (Statham, 1996).

The project has employed a number of different research methods, and took place in three stages.

**Stage one** took place in late 1992/early 1993, approximately one year after the implementation of the Children Act. The purpose of the first stage was to monitor how the Act had been initially implemented. It was a 'mapping exercise' against which to measure the evolving impact of the Act over time. It involved visits by members of the research team to a range of local authority officers involved with services for young children who were interviewed using a semi-structured interview schedule. The findings of this first stage are reported in Bull et al. (1994a).

Stages two and three of the project were concerned mainly with assessing the impact of the Act on day care services, around three years after its implementation. **Stage two** took place between January and May 1994. It comprised:

- case studies around the themes of provision, co-ordination and regulation in a small number of contrasting local authorities (referred to as the 'case studies'). A full report of this element of the research is provided in Bull et al. (1994b);
- a national survey of day care providers in the private and voluntary sectors selected from local authority registers of independent day care services (referred to as the 'service providers survey'). A full report of the survey is provided in Moss et al. (1995);
- a written request to all local authorities for any surveys undertaken of parents' views about services for young children.

**Stage three** involved return visits, in the winter of 1994/95, to the local authorities visited in stage one, where the range of respondents was widened to include local authority staff involved in registration, inspection and support (hereafter referred to as regulation managers, regulation officers and support officers) and representatives of the voluntary sector from a selected number of agencies or groups, in order to make a fuller assessment of the impact of the Act in its third year of implementation.

The range and number of respondents – local authority staff, providers and representatives of voluntary groups – included in each stage of the research and the methods used are summarised in box 1.2.

The work at all three stages was focused on a representative national sample of English local authorities. The sampling strategy was to randomly select one in six of all authorities, stratified by local authority type, giving a total sample of 18 authorities for the first stage, and, due to the withdrawal of one local authority from the study, 17 local authorities in the second and third stages. This sampling strategy ensured that a range of local authority types was included, from densely populated inner city or metropolitan areas to rural districts. It also ensured that the results of the study could, in principle, be generalised to provide a national picture.

**Box 1.2**

**How the research was carried out**

- Interviews with 85 key local authority officers concerned with services for young children, in social services, education and leisure departments in 18 sample local authorities: at end of first year of implementation (Bull et al., 1994a).
- Case studies in a sub-group of six local authorities on the themes of regulation, coordination and provision, involving further interviews with local authority officers, voluntary sector groups and some providers: between second and third year of implementation (Bull et al., 1994b).
- A survey of 425 independent day care providers randomly selected from lists of registered provision in 17 sample local authorities; between second and third year of implementation (Moss et al., 1995).
- The collection from all English local authorities of any surveys used to obtain parental views of services, between the second and third year of implementation.

- Follow up interviews with 17 key officers in the sample authorities, at end of third year of implementation.

- Interviews with 78 local authority staff involved with the registration, inspection and support of private day care services, including managers and field staff, from 17 sample local authorities, at end of third year of implementation.

- Personal or telephone interviews with representatives from selected voluntary sector agencies, including organisations representing independent sector providers (e.g., the PLA, NCMA, KCN), local early years forums, and a relevant disability organisation and minority ethnic group in each of the 17 sample local authorities, at end of third year of implementation.

### Issues in evaluating the Act

The research reported in this book has been concerned with evaluating the impact of the Children Act on services for young children, especially day care services for children aged under five, and central to this evaluation has been the assessment of the Act against the objectives it outlined for services at the time of implementation. However, making a precise evaluation is difficult, if not impossible, for a number of reasons:

- The Act's *objectives are not always clearly articulated* – for example, is the purpose of regulation raising quality or maintaining minimum standards? The Department of Health's view is that regulation under the Act is intended to achieve both objectives (personal communication). But the Act itself says nothing about the objectives of regulation. Nor does Guidance include quality in the four functions it ascribes to the regulatory process – it refers to ensuring 'acceptable standards' – although it goes on to say that 'registration has to be a positive process, there to help the setting up of good quality services' (cf. Guidance, para. 4.9). Additionally, some of the objectives originally contained in the Act and Guidance have been qualified over time, particularly in the light of Circular LAC (93)1.

- There are *many gaps in knowledge about the situation that existed in relation to day care services before the Act*. For example, we have no baseline data about the standards in day care services before the new regulation regime; the extent and nature of support and training offered to providers; and levels of provision for children in need. It is therefore difficult to make precise pre- and post-Act comparisons.

- Despite this lack of precise knowledge of pre-Act conditions, it is clear that *local authorities were at very different points* – of organisation, philosophy and provision of services – when the Act was introduced; which as McQuail and Pugh (1995: 118) also note 'complicates the task of distinguishing between different aspects of performance'.
- The *wide range of contextual factors* to which we have already referred makes it difficult to distinguish what results from the Act, from other factors or from the interaction between the Act and these factors.

Because of the difficulties involved in evaluating the outcomes of the Act, the approach to evaluating the Act which we have adopted is that of a process evaluation, described by Littlewood (1994: 6) as follows:

> *process evaluation concentrates on assessing how a policy is put into practice, what happens on the ground and how this relates to how the policy is meant to work.*

The following chapters are structured around the main duties and powers in relation to day care services given to local authorities in the Children Act: provision, co-ordination, regulation, and support for services. Each chapter begins by reviewing the Act and introducing some debates about its particular theme; this is followed with a review of where matters had got to three years after implementation and an evaluation of the Act's impact; each chapter concludes by listing a number of lessons arising from the research. In consideration of the Act's support for the principle of partnership with parents, a chapter which considers the ways in which local authorities have attempted to seek parents' views is also included. A full list of publications arising from the studies conducted in England and Wales is included in Appendix 1.

CHAPTER

# 2 Provision of Services for Young Children

**Claire Cameron**

## Background

The Children Act had specific and limited objectives in the area of service provision for young children. The Act was largely concerned with day care rather than education services, and within day care it reaffirmed the existing policy of public provision only in certain cases defined by health or welfare need. For the most part, parents remain responsible for funding day care through paying fees for services in the private and voluntary sector. Thus the traditional separation of provision of day care for welfare purposes and general day care provision is retained, at least conceptually, although the Act and Guidance make suggestions about overcoming this separation in practice. The Act and Guidance also make some suggestions designed to improve the ways in which services are delivered in local authority areas.

Objectives for provision contained in the Children Act include:

- a duty to provide a range and level of services appropriate to children 'in need', including a duty to provide family centres (the only type of day care provision specified);
- a duty to facilitate such provision by the voluntary sector and others as the local authority sees fit;
- a duty to provide day care services for children 'in need' under the age of five, after school and in school holidays for children 'in need' over the age of five;
- a power to provide day care services for children not 'in need'.

In addition, local authorities are required to:

- publish information about day care for parents;
- have regard to the racial groups to which children 'in need' belong.

Guidance interprets the Act by emphasising:

- the need for local authorities to have an agreed policies for discharging their duty to provide day care for children 'in need';
- encouragement to use and develop the private and voluntary sector both in general and for children 'in need';
- respect for the views of parents and children;
- the need for a variety of day care services in order for parents to be able to exercise choice about the type and location of the day care service.

Finally, Circular LAC (93)1 emphasised the desirability of expansion of general day care services in the private and voluntary sectors.

**The Wider Debate**

The hallmark of day care provision in Britain is diversity. As noted in chapter 1, services for young children embrace a wide range of types, such as home-based child minding and centre-based playgroups and day nurseries. Another dimension of diversity in day care services is the multitude of different organisations and associations which run the services, as well as those run by individuals. Against this fragmented background of day care, nearly all of which is in the private and voluntary sector, there are also nursery education services in the public sector[2], which obviously serves an overlapping age group of children. Alongside this range of services, the distribution of day care and early education is both uneven and limited (Moss and Owen 1989; Owen and Moss 1989), so the plethora of types does not guarantee a choice of services to the parent in need of day care for their pre-school child.

The question arises as to whether this diversity is the product of day care 'policy', or whether it is only in retrospect that it is possible to identify the government's policy through an accumulation of documents such as government reports. Certainly there has been no policy review of day care or early years provision on a national basis. But government clearly applauds the principle of diversity as a source of strength in services for young children (e.g. Hansard, 18 January 1989, 397–8), although this may be a *post hoc* approval of the existing situation.

2. Such as nursery schools and classes, and many four year olds are admitted to reception classes of infant schools.

However, using government circulars as a guide to policy, it is possible to see that there is a longstanding policy for the provision of day care which limits public responsibility to those children whose welfare is a cause for concern, or whose mothers are 'constrained into having to go out to work' (MoH Circular 37/68). Otherwise the government believes that parents are responsible for day care services as they are the ones to make the arrangements, 'including financial arrangements, for the day care of pre-school age children' (Education Select Committee, 1989:197). Policy for day care, up to the enactment of the Children Act, is largely residual in remit and restrictive in its ambitions. One result of historically low levels of public provision is that services for young children in Britain are a disparate collection of private, public and voluntary sector funded services serving children of different age groups, and with overlapping purposes embracing education, care and welfare.

Similarly, public policy on the provision of education for children aged under five, such as nursery schooling, is discretionary (Education Select Committee, 1989:156) and as a result, there is more nursery education in metropolitan and London authorities than in county councils (Statham et al., 1990). Further there is a relationship between the distribution of playgroups and that of nursery education, so that 'playgroups are most commonly found in local authorities with relatively few nursery education places, and vice versa' (Statham et al., 1990: 28). Nursery education provides a free, generally accessible, non-stigmatising service open to all children, and as such forms a significant element of policies on access to services for young children adopted by local authorities. In contrast, local authorities have rarely aspired to make day care services open to all children under five.

Beyond the role of local authorities in providing services for young children, there have been policy initiatives aimed at the expansion of the supply of services for young children from within the voluntary and private sectors. Examples of this include government sponsored child care subsidies for women employed on lower incomes (Duncan et al., 1995), and employer supported child care, such as workplace nurseries or a voucher scheme for employees to redeem against their own paid arrangements (Moss, 1992).

The initiative offering perhaps the most significant impact on both day care and early education services is the proposed voucher scheme for subsidising a 'pre-school place' within day care or education services for four year olds, subject to meeting certain educational criteria (Shephard, 1995).

The desirability of expanding early education had been recommended in several high profile reports (National Commission on Education, 1993; Ball, C.,1994). These reports drew on American research (e.g., Schweinhart and Weikart, 1993), which suggested that there were strong economic arguments for extending nursery education. The voucher scheme endorses maintained and private sector educational provision, and plans to stimulate new provision in the private and voluntary sector. Specifically, it recognises an educational role for playgroups and day nurseries in the private and voluntary sector (Shephard, 1995).

Early concerns about the scheme expressed by the voluntary sector include the details of the financial and administrative arrangements, and the implications that a focus on provision for four years olds will have on other children under five receiving a day care service (National Early Years Network Briefing, August 1995; Coordinate, March 1996).

Lastly, as the Children Act focuses on provision for children in 'need', the concept of need requires some consideration. Social need is a 'notoriously slippery concept' for which there are varying interpretations, such as 'professionally defined need', 'consumer demand' and 'shortfall' (Smith, 1990). The Children Act emphasises children's health and behaviour as a guide to defining 'in need' (section 17), which suggests a reliance on professional definitions to assess eligibility for publicly-funded day care services. The Act also gives greater emphasis to the provision of day care services, and in particular, family centres, than contained in previous legislation, explicitly identifying these services as part of 'family support services' (Part III). Aldgate et al. argue that section 17 of the Children Act 'represents a three-dimensional change in concept from earlier legislation'. Firstly, service delivery, rather than social work advice and counselling, is emphasised; secondly, the concept of 'family support' and 'promotion of welfare' is deployed rather than the narrower 'prevention of reception into care'; and thirdly, the use of 'in need' focuses attention on a specific group of children to whom help should be directed (Aldgate et al., 1994: 2).

There is a potential tension between the use of a professionally-led assessment process based on criteria relating to a child's health and welfare, and a general expansion of access to day care services on grounds of need based on social disadvantage, for example. For children in their early years at least, the use of the term 'in need' appears designed to continue the long-held policy of limited public provision of day care services, while at the same time addressing recommendations in government reports preceding the Children Act (e.g., DHSS, 1985; DoH, 1987) for a greater use of general services, including day care, to help families look after their children.

In conclusion, the wider debate about the provision of services for young children focuses on the means of delivering an expansion of day care services, and most recently early education, in the private and voluntary sector. The Children Act has contributed to the debate by recommending ways of providing services, particularly for children 'in need', with an emphasis on family centres and the use of independent sector provision.

## Implementation Three Years After the Act

Data considered in this chapter derive from follow-up interviews at the third stage with a sample of 17 local authority policy officers, and where relevant from representatives of various concerned voluntary organisations. Such representative organisations were not always available in each local authority, and had widely differing experiences. Their comments have been selected and included to illustrate points, rather than to offer a representative view.

*Early years policies and delivery*

Local authorities began their implementation of the Children Act from widely varying points in the level of provision, and in the existence of organisational structures and dedicated policy officer time to develop and implement policies. At one extreme, some local authorities had a longstanding policy commitment to provide services for young children on a universal basis, while at the other, some local authorities had no written policy for, and little provision of, day care or early years education services. The final stage of this study demonstrated that such variations still existed three years after the implementation of the Act, although even where there was no written policy, developments in the provision of services had occurred. Formal policy was not necessary, in other words, for changes in the delivery of services.

Broadly speaking, the local authorities in this sample demonstrated three types of policy. Firstly, there was a group of authorities which had broad *early years* policies, covering day care and education, with a high level of existing nursery education and a high level of commitment to developing day care provision in the private and voluntary sector. Decision making tended to be done on a corporate basis, with ideally a significant formal input from representatives of the private and voluntary sector. The emphasis in these authorities was on providing services directly, with an aim to have services universally accessible, which usually meant part-time nursery education for all three and four year olds. Eight authorities in the sample fell into the broad 'early years policies' group, though not all of them included the independent sector in policy making.

Secondly, there were authorities with *day care* policies (separate from education policies), where the focus was on providing services for children 'in need', and on developing other services (such as full-time day care, or out of school services) in 'partnership' with other agencies, such as the voluntary sector, and government agencies such as the TECs. Decision making here tended to be led by social services departments, with consultations with the private and voluntary sector and other local authority departments. Five local authorities had such a policy.

Thirdly, there was a group of four local authorities with no written policy for day care or early years. These authorities generally had a low level of existing day care and nursery education services, little or no dedicated policy officer time to progress implementation of the Act and no joint decision-making structures between social services and other local authority departments.

Two points about these groups need mentioning. First, the relationship between policy and existing provision was not always predictable. High levels of existing early years provision did not necessarily mean that policies were constructed on a corporate basis or at least in part, jointly between social services and other local authority departments. Three local authorities with high levels of provision located their policy making within social services departments, and two of these had 'universal' access as their aspiration. Second, half the local authorities in the *early years policy* group did not wish to restrict themselves to providing services directly. They were also committed to developing an 'enabling' role with other local organisations. This meant considerable efforts had gone into developing relationships with the voluntary sector, both by involving them in decision making, and in providing grant aid to private and voluntary sector groups.

This method of grouping local authority policies relies on *inclusiveness*, or coherence of policies across all services for young children. Another way of grouping the various policy approaches to early years is to consider how local authorities viewed their new 'provider' responsibilities in the Children Act. The main responsibilities included here are those to provide, and to monitor the need for, services for children 'in need', and those to promote access to services for children not 'in need'. The Act encouraged a 'partnership' approach to the development of provision within the private and voluntary sector, so this is a significant element in grouping policies and approaches under the new legislation. This method produces groups of local authorities which have been termed the *traditionalists*, the *enablers* and the *minimalists* in this chapter.

*Traditionalists* comprise the five authorities with a strong history of providing early education and day care services, usually with the aim of universal access to the services, from within separate departments. Two authorities within this group found the requirement to provide for children 'in need' under the Act initially difficult to reconcile with their aim of universal access, and have viewed the Act as something to be accommodated within their existing framework, rather than providing an opportunity to pursue new methods of delivering services.

*Enablers* are the seven authorities who, while having high levels of their own provision, had sought to develop services further in 'partnership' with other agencies. 'Partnership' is here taken to include providing grant aid to the independent sector, the participation of these sectors in policy making, and funding service development posts within the local authority. Three of the authorities in this group pursued such methods before the implementation of the Children Act, and for four, the policy was reinvigorated in the light of the Act. This is the group where the Act is most likely to have had an impact on early years provision.

Lastly, *minimalists* are those five authorities with low levels of own service provision, who viewed the legislation in the area of provision for under eights as largely presenting duties to provide some family support services for children 'in need'. These included the four local authorities with no written policy for day care or early years.

Before leaving these models of policy, it is worth briefly mentioning the organisational structures for decision making for early years (an issue explored in greater detail in the next chapter). Some authorities had integrated services, where the traditional split between day care and education services had been overcome by creating a separate department, or unit within a department. Other authorities had developed structures for decision making on early years issues that were located at least partly outside social services departments. In this sample, there were three authorities which had pursued 'integration', and six that had adopted a corporate or more co-ordinated approach. Neither method of organisation entirely predicted authorities' membership of the groupings outlined here, except that all but one of those adopting a corporate/co-ordinated approach were in the 'enabler' group.

Examples of the structures included an *Early Years Development Officer*, reporting to an Early Years Sub-Committee (Policy Committee) and the Chief Executives Department; a *Young Children's Service*, reporting to the Young Children's Sub-Committee and the Education Department; and an *Under Eights Section*, reporting to an Under-8s Sub-Committee, and the Community Education Department. All of the six co-ordinated authorities had dedicated policy officer time to develop policies and implement the legislation, in contrast to the minimalists and the traditionalists, where the majority of authorities did not have such a resource.

**Box 2.1**

**An example of an enabler authority**

A metropolitan authority with above-average levels of nursery education and playgroups, and medium levels of childminders and day nurseries (both local authority and registered), this authority has integrated its policy and provision for early years under one department. In addition, the building which houses regulation officers and policy officers also offers office space to the key voluntary sector organisations in the city which enables direct liaison. The authority has constructed 'ward profiles' of early years provision throughout the city. This means there is a thorough knowledge of where the provision is situated and helps decide where future provision should be located. There are a number of development initiatives throughout the city such as training packages for all childcare workers; a pilot scheme for a childminders' business initiative; and a sponsored childminder scheme for supporting childminders looking after children 'in need'.

**Resources**

Policy officer respondents were asked about changes in resources during the period of implementation of the Children Act. Specifically they were asked whether any audit of spending on children aged under eight had been completed, whether this extended across departments, and whether there had been any changes in the amount spent since the Children Act was introduced in three areas: providing services, regulating services and training and support for day care workers.

This is an extremely complex area for two reasons. Firstly, the demarcation of 'children under eight' is a new category and not all expenditure on provision can be separated out according to this age group. The chief example is primary education, which forms a considerable proportion of total spending on children aged under eight, but is grouped under headings related to the institution rather than the age group. Thus the cost of schools are counted rather than cost per child. The second reason is that there is no consistent method of accounting for expenditure across local authorities. Thus while one local authority could give an accurate assessment covering public and voluntary sector spending, for example, another could give figures relating only to grant-aid to voluntary groups, or in some cases no figures at all. Comparisons, therefore, are more or less impossible.

Our experience of the impossibility of getting comprehensive, comparable and longitudinal information on resources mirrors the experience of a recent National Children's Bureau study of 11 local authorities:

> *There was also surprisingly inadequate financial information available from the local authorities, so that it was impossible to detect any trends across all authorities. It was also not possible to compare expenditure on all services for under fives over the five year period, as there was no integrated financial information (McQuail and Pugh, 1995: 3)*

The perception of policy officer respondents, on the whole, was of an increase in the amount spent on services for young children since the Children Act. There was more likely to have been an increase in resources for regulating services, and least likely to have been an increase in resources for training and support of day care workers (see also chapters 4 and 5). Eleven local authorities reported an increase in resources for providing services, but in four of these the increase was attributed to spending in nursery education rather than the Children Act.

*Children 'in need'*

There is a specific but general duty for local authorities to provide day care services for children 'in need' within their area, and to have regard to the 'different racial groups' to which the children belong (s.17 and Schedule 2 para.11). In addition there is a duty to identify the extent of need and then make decisions on the priorities for service provision in their area (s.17). While the Children Act gives a broad definition of 'in need', referring to the impairment of the health and behaviour of individual children, and children who are disabled, it is left to local authorities to provide a more precise definition of the term.

**Table 2.1: Summary of policy officer responses to question of changes in resources since the Children Act**

| N=17 | Increase in spending on provision of services | Increase in spending on regulation of services | Increase in spending on training and support of day care workers |
|---|---|---|---|
| | 11 | 14 | 6 |

The first stage of this study (Bull et al., 1994a) reported that local definitions of need tended to prioritise 'need' in terms of statutory responsibilities held by the local authority. Thus children on the Child Protection Register or subject to Care Orders would have a more immediate claim on services than children living in other circumstances. This finding has been confirmed by other studies (DoH, 1994; Aldgate et al., 1994; Audit Commission, 1994). A second finding was that local authorities tended to use an individual assessment process to identify and classify children 'in need', rather than identify groups or areas likely to be 'in need' and target service provision accordingly. In addition in some areas the concept of 'in need' was resisted, and the authorities preferred to make services available on a universal basis.

In the second and third stages of the study it was apparent that local authorities were even more likely to be using an individual assessment of 'need' than one based on geographical areas or socio-economic groups. However, three local authorities were trying to combine both methods of identification, individual and area-based, through local planning processes and computer-based information systems with the idea of more effectively targeting resources for service development.

*Changes in service provision for children 'in need'*

One local authority was unable to provide a respondent equipped to answer questions on provision for children 'in need' and so the number of authorities in the sample for this section is 16.

The measures to provide services within the Children Act gave local authorities an opportunity to 'ensure that a range of services is available..[and] in addition to day care provision for pre-school and school age children it is likely that a range of services designed to support and improve the strengths and skills of parents...will be required' (DoH 1991: para. 2.11). Unlike previous legislation, the Act specifies a particular form of support; family centres for the purposes of 'occupational, social, cultural or recreational activities or advice' (ibid: para. 9, Schedule 2). Another innovation in this area was to include children with disabilities within the definition of children 'in need'.

There are three main ways local authorities can meet their duty to provide services. One is to provide 'directly', that is where the authority owns and manages the facility such as a day nursery or family centre; another is a 'partnership' model, where the local authority and a voluntary agency such as a children's charity (e.g. Barnados, NCH, Save the Children) enter into some joint arrangement to run the facility; and a third is 'sponsorship', where a local authority 'places and pays for' a child to attend a general day care service such as a childminder or playgroup. Particular forms of provision may be more or less appropriate in particular kinds of environment (Statham and Cameron, 1994). Nearly all authorities used all three methods of delivering services, although the mix varied. All authorities had at least one day nursery or family centre, and all the enablers employed the 'partnership' model to extend their family centre provision, as did half of the traditionalists and minimalists. It can be seen from table 2.2 that sponsorship of childminders was used by all authorities, but sponsorship of other services in the private and voluntary sector tailed off quite rapidly, with only ten using day nurseries and six sponsoring places in family centres. Enabler and minimalist authorities were more likely to use a range of services in the private and voluntary sector than the traditionalists. Six of the seven enablers, and four of the five minimalists reported using four or more types of private and voluntary sector service.

There was little change in the provision of services since the Children Act was implemented. New service development was often accompanied by concurrent cutbacks in services. Six local authorities had new family centres or had extended the roles of their family centres, and three had new day nurseries or early years centres. However, five of these nine authorities had also cut back their centre-based provision, and a further two authorities had implemented cuts without any expansion. Three authorities had developed partnership family centres; one of these was a resource centre for children with disabilities. Four local authorities had extended their use of sponsorship of day care places in a range of settings.

**Table 2.2: Summary of use of different forms of provision for children 'in need'**

| N = 16 | Direct provision | Partnership | Sponsorship |
|---|---|---|---|
| | 13 | 10 | 16 – Childminders |
| | | | 13 – Playgroups |
| | | | 10 – Day nurseries |
| | | | 8 – Holiday play schemes |
| | | | 7 – Out-of-school schemes |
| | | | 6 – Family centres |

However, beyond this rather limited picture, some local authorities described innovative schemes for extending and developing provision for children 'in need', which included working across agencies and imaginative ways of working in a financially restrictive climate. Some examples include:

- joint funded (education and social services) peripatetic nursery officer for children with disabilities;
- joint funded (PPA, health authority and social services) sponsorship scheme for PPA member playgroups;
- redistribution of staff to achieve three new 'early years teams' to develop community based services in areas of disadvantage;
- two childminder support schemes within a city with employed support staff and a budget to provide free places.

*Sponsorship and the views of the voluntary sector*

The Children Act and Guidance encouraged the use of private and voluntary services for children 'in need', but, as has been argued elsewhere (Cameron and Statham, forthcoming), this can present difficulties for service providers themselves. Voluntary sector organisations were asked about their perception of the use of their services for children 'in need'. While some had no experience of this, for those that did a number of general issues were raised. These concerned the support and training available to day care providers, the unequal relationship between the local authority and the voluntary sector and the financial pressures on voluntary sector groups.

The comments of the voluntary sector (see box 2.2 for some examples of these comments) illustrate both the promise and the problems of involving childminders and playgroups in looking after children 'in need'. On the one hand, voluntary sector facilities are very well placed to care for children in their local area, and it seems that since the Children Act, more services have been asked to do this. But conversely, the work brings additional pressures, such as fundraising for equipment, or more stretched support services and networks. The picture emerging is one of the private and voluntary sector being under intense pressure, and unsure of its means of influencing local authority decision making. Some of these issues are also discussed in chapters 4 and 5.

**Box 2.2**

**Comments from voluntary organisations**

- 'More is pushed our way. Social workers see the need for day care and after-school places and are leaning on services, but are not providing resources. They have reduced the amount paid to PPA support network, so much so that field workers can only visit in areas of high need. Many groups are left on their own. Support networks are being eaten away – and this is a very important aspect of provision for children 'in need''.

- 'The cut of money for children 'in need' has been complete. Unless on the 'at risk' register children won't qualify for help. So if a child needs one to one or equipment the playgroups have to raise funds themselves'.

- 'In some cases children 'in need' are taken out of playgroups and put in centres – not a good thing. Needs can be met by the voluntary sector but are generally not at present. The definition of 'in need' is ambiguous. There are children 'in need' in the voluntary sector – more behavioural/ emotional. The voluntary sector is left with these children without extra resources or recognition. The attitude of the local authority to the voluntary sector is 'we're in charge''.

- 'The local authority will approach us for a place on the grounds of a child being at risk or abused rather than low income or single parent. We can't approach them. We would like the government to give us money to be able to offer sponsored places or less expensive care, rather than the local authority'.

- 'Since the Children Act we tend to get more referrals and do more preventative work'.
- 'Childminders could be used more effectively for children in need with the right support and training. Social services departments haven't really thought about this. I put a proposal for a community childminding scheme to committee. It was rejected – I don't know why. There may be ways of doing it at a more local level'.

*Planning and monitoring for children 'in need'*

One of the difficulties in precise measurement of changes in service provision for children 'in need' is the general absence of systems for planning and monitoring both services and the population of children who use the services. Guidance emphasised the importance of planning and monitoring to enable effective use of services by those 'in need'. It states that local authorities should both identify the extent of need among the population in their areas and 'evaluate and monitor the availability' of services such as day care (DoH, 1991: para. 2.12).

This study suggests that at the time of final stage interviews local authorities were having difficulty making progress with these responsibilities. In general few local authorities were able to estimate the numbers of children 'in need', and few had appropriate systems in place to monitor the number and characteristics of children 'in need' using a day care service or in need of, and waiting for, a day care service.

The progress made with these areas of responsibility was spread across all three 'policy types' represented in this sample. Of the four local authorities who could estimate the numbers of children 'in need', two were from the enabler group, and two were minimalists. Of the eight authorities who were establishing systems for tracking the number of children 'in need' receiving a day care service, two were traditionalist, and there were three each from the other two groups. A more detailed profile of the characteristics of the placement was being developed in two traditionalist, two enabler and one minimalist local authority.

**Table 2.3: Summary of progress of sample local authorities in estimating numbers and monitoring the profile of children aged under eight 'in need'**

| LAs N = 16 | Estimates Completed | | Monitoring Underway | | |
|---|---|---|---|---|---|
| | Total number of children 'in need' | Total number of children under eight 'in need' | Known number 'in need' receiving day care service | Known why placed; what type; duration of placement | Know size of waiting list |
| YES | 4 | 0 | 8[1] | 5[2] | 4 |
| NO | 12 | 16 | 8 | 11 | 12 |

[1] includes one where system being introduced; one where numbers known only in own provision

[2] includes three where being introduced; two where information known locally but not centrally

Various difficulties with the planning and monitoring tasks were mentioned by respondents. One policy officer referred to a problematic relationship between knowing the extent of need and responsibility for meeting that need: 'local authorities are hard pressed to meet known need, without extending our responsibility to unknown need'. Another problem among those local authorities trying to estimate the extent of need is that of the different ways data are compiled. For example while the 1991 Census provides comprehensive information, it is not easy to extract information about children aged under eight. One respondent said they had tried to estimate the extent of known need but 'we had such problems we had to give it up'.

Those authorities that had managed to estimate numbers had done so on the basis of collating estimates for a range of key indicators. One authority gave examples of indicators which included numbers of refugee children, numbers of children with special educational needs, the numbers of children with disabilities and known to have special health needs; and those 'looked after' by the local authority and on the child protection register. Other respondents mentioned indicators deriving from social security benefits, such as recipients of free school meals or housing benefit as the basis for estimating 'in need' numbers.

There appeared to be few, if any, common factors among those authorities who had made progress with the monitoring duties under the Children Act. One factor could be the dedicated policy officer time available to progress information systems. Two of the authorities who had made progress were such authorities, but others with policy officer time had not made similar progress and others who had made progress did not appear to have policy time available. Another factor could be the physical size of the local authority. It tends to be easier to set up new information systems in smaller areas, where the data to be collected are perhaps more manageable and the personnel involved are likely to be in regular contact with each other. Three of the authorities who had made progress were small metropolitan or London boroughs, but one was a large county and one a small outer London borough. But again, other small authorities had not made progress, and in at least two of the metropolitan areas the sheer scale of the data collection exercise were impressive. A third possible explanation is that insufficient time has elapsed since the passage of the Act to enable the bulk of the local authorities to make progress with these new and difficult tasks.

Another aspect of monitoring is the monitoring of spending. In an earlier publication we argued that

> *systems for tracking the number and cost of children in need and with special needs in day care need to be established....This will enable [local authorities] to have a better idea of the overall needs for the development of the service. A start could be made by separating day care sponsorship budgets [from other budgets] (Bull et al., 1994b)*

This was also recommended by the Audit Commission (1994: 44). In this stage of the study we asked policy officers whether they had a specific budget for paying for day care for children 'in need', or whether it was absorbed into the general section 17 (family support) budget. Nine local authorities said they had a specific budget and seven did not. Five of these nine authorities fell into the enabler group, and two each in the traditionalist and minimalist. In almost all cases these budgets were held by social services area managers or their equivalents.

*Children with disabilities*

One area of services for children 'in need' appeared to fare better than the rest. This was children with disabilities. From the perspective of local authority policy officers, the position for children with disabilities had markedly improved since the introduction of the Children Act. The duty to introduce a joint health authority/social services register of children with disabilities has in the words of one respondent

> *highlighted their needs. We've used that and the children 'in need' process to strengthen our hand in getting resources.*

Fourteen authorities had, or were well into the process of, establishing their registers. Fourteen authorities had integrated services for children with disabilities into general children and families work, twelve of these since the implementation of the Act. Three local authorities, all of whom were in the enabler group, stood out in their comments on progress in this area.

In one authority 'maximum integration' was energetically pursued as a policy in all early years establishments, with, for example, reserved places within a day nursery. However, when asked about the impact of the Act in this area, the respondent said

> *there was a huge drift towards integration anyway. The Children Act has given the impetus to work more closely [with other agencies and departments].*

In the second authority to stand out the respondent commented on

> *a lot of progress in day care services, integrating disabled children into ordinary day care services. There are pockets of good practice. Also [there is] a 'disability day care' budget of £12,000 to make packages to help keep disabled children in the community, and more resources for opportunity playgroups.*

In the third authority, the attention given to the issue by one services development manager was seen to have been effective. Many local authority services were not accessible to the non-ambulant, but many had children with learning difficulties, and

> *the culture is slowly beginning to change. We see children with disabilities as part of our responsibility, within mainstream provision. We are not there yet, but getting there. The culture of inclusion is being pushed in nurseries.*

Representatives of voluntary organisations concerned with children with disabilities were not so overwhelmingly positive about the position for children with disabilities. Some made comments that illuminated vividly both progress and problems. One said:

> *The Children Act emphasis on children 'in need' and children with disabilities has enabled a doubling of care staff and care hours to extend [respite care] service to children. It has been stimulating a range of services... and looked at children with disabilities as a specific group for the*

*first time. The new team has given parents and children a focus...They've achieved a lot in a short space of time.*

But another said:

*Cutbacks in schools have meant there is some discrimination against children with disabilities. School are less willing to take children with special needs. There is less flexibility in provision. [But] respite care [day and overnight] is changing – becoming more flexible and responsive. There is not enough support for children with disabilities going into playgroups in rural areas. Parents have campaigned for support from the education department, now the local authority is agreeing to provide some more support.*

One possible explanation for this divergence of opinion is that the policy officer respondents, who were primarily from within social services departments, viewed the progress with services for children with disabilities as more rapid because the responsibilities were relatively new, whereas those working within the voluntary sector have often been campaigning for improvements in services for a longer time.

*Changes in service provision for all children*

The Children Act gave local authorities a power to provide day care for children not 'in need', but Guidance pointed out that 'public funds' are unlikely to 'be sufficient to provide day care for all parents who wish to use such a service' (DoH 1991: para 4.8). Data from this study suggested that it was indeed difficult to pursue this method of expanding provision. One local authority's service plan put the position as: 'Local authorities are also empowered to offer [day care and supervised activities] to children not in need but most [including this one] have insufficient resources to do so'.

Instead Guidance suggested that local authorities, in 'consultation with other departments and interests', might wish to set up a day care service for a wide range of children in areas of multiple disadvantage, or where there is a need to upgrade a locality, or to encourage other organisations to set up facilities (DoH 1991: para 4.8). Beyond these suggestions for specific models of day care, Circular LAC (93)1 explicitly encouraged an expansion of services within the private and voluntary sectors when it said 'the Government is concerned to encourage the expansion of day care facilities...[which is] extremely desirable'.

The service providers' survey made clear the difficulties of matching demand within the current framework of service types and their availability. Playgroups and many childminders are available for a limited number of hours per week, and not during the school holidays. Other childminders may be more flexible and offer before and after school care, and day nurseries are generally open all year, but only between set hours. Despite this, many providers reported vacancies and difficulties filling places, particularly among nurseries, and many reported holding a waiting list of children old enough to start (Moss et al., 1995). The Children Act, however, did not address these structural difficulties with the provision as organised at present. Rather, through the emphasis on market solutions and enabling the private and voluntary sector to flourish, the Act and the Circular gives a higher priority to the principle of 'diversity' of service types and availability.

The Act and Guidance did provide two means of improving access to the existing day care services. The first is the duty to publish information about day care services (Schedule 2 para. 1), and the second is a good practice recommendation in Guidance to promote equal opportunities policies and practice (DoH, 1991: paras. 6.10, 6.11).

*Information services*

The Act requires local authorities to publish information about the services they provide and, where appropriate, those provided by other organisations, and Guidance suggests possible methods by which this may be done (ibid: para. 5.11). One method is to publish a directory of services; another is to run or enable a specialist child care information service in the locality, perhaps run on a partnership basis with the voluntary sector, employers, the private day care sector and the local authority (ibid: para. 5.12).

Data from this study suggested that progress in the area of information services was generally limited, with one or two exceptions. Some authorities where an information service already existed have improved it; others have recognised the need for a database, and/or have published a directory. The policy officer respondents were asked how they enable parents to find out about services for young children; the main way reported was still through social services area offices and day care officers who hold lists of registered provision to be sent out on request. Methods of supplying information about services for young children reported by local authority officers included:

- Lists of registered provision sent out by area social services offices.
- Leaflets distributed via local authority day nurseries.
- Advice in person at specific times from a day care officer ('surgery').
- Advice over the telephone at specific times from a day care officer ('duty system').
- Computer information service in libraries, other public buildings.
- Directory of local services.
- 'One stop' child care information service.

Three 'levels' of information service to parents can be discerned. The first level is for the social services department to send out lists of registered providers on request. The second level is to send out lists and publish a directory and advisory or information leaflets, and to distribute these widely. Seven of 17 local authorities used these methods. The third level is to run a comprehensive child care information service, where parents can discuss child care plans with an advisor, either in person or on the telephone, where information about vacancies and special facilities are recorded and day care facilities are promoted. This 'one stop' service can be run by the local authority, by a voluntary organisation grant-aided by the local authority, or by an independent consortium of interested agencies. Ten local authorities reported having some kind of 'one stop' service, four of these run by voluntary organisations, and six by the local authority. None of these had been set up in the light of the Children Act's recommendations. Not all of the 'one stop' services were available across the entire local authority. For example, one 'partnership' model of information service was dependent on the subscription of large employers and operated in mainly urban areas of the county. There was no systematic association between policy 'types' and style of information services. As with monitoring duties, this may be because insufficient time since implementation has elapsed for substantial progress towards the establishment of a comprehensive information service.

Policy officer respondents were asked about any ways in which non-English speaking parents might find out about services for young children. Six local authorities reported having some way for non-English speakers to access information. Typically this was a written introduction or summary to a directory available in languages commonly spoken in the local authority area, which referred to an interpreter service.

Two representatives of organisations providing services for minority ethnic children illustrated difficulties that can arise in gaining access to information. In one, an authority with a child care information shop, the respondent said the service was advertised in council leaflets, that the 'shop front' image was helpful, and that a quarterly newsletter was circulated to parents and organisations (for a nominal fee) and was printed in several languages. But, she continued

> *I'm not so sure people do take part in practice. A lot of Muslim parents like their children to go to nurseries and creches where they can speak their own language. Access is not always there. The financial constraints are a big part of it. Unless the service is free and on your doorstep – people need things there for all ages and stages.*

In another authority, with no information service or strategy, a respondent said information was not accessible

> *unless [a mother is] experienced. We provide an information system here. We know childminders who may be able to help.*

These experiences of difficulty gaining access to information are likely to be reflected in difficulty gaining access to services. This point will be considered below.

Various difficulties with the duty to publish information were noted by policy officer respondents. Firstly, written information such as leaflets and directories quickly become out of date. Secondly, the use made of any leaflets is difficult to monitor. Directories, we were told, are expensive and time consuming to compile and maintain. Computer held databases hold more promise but are similarly time consuming to compile, and need to be widely accessible and regularly updated. One county council in our sample employed an information officer whose duties included providing lists of provision tailored according to parents needs, such as day care available *en route* to their workplace from home. This service was also accessible via a general computer information service held in libraries and other public buildings.

*Equal opportunities*

Guidance makes a good practice recommendation that people working with young children should enable them to 'develop positive attitudes to differences of race, culture and language and differences of gender', and that local authorities should have 'approved equal opportunities policies'. They should collate data on the ethnic origins of the local population, and ensure that 'services operate in a non-discriminatory way' (DoH 1991: paras 6.10, 6.11). The emphasis is on ethnicity and race; gender issues are given only a minor mention. Disability issues are not specifically mentioned under this heading in the Guidance, but as the integration of children with a disability is a seen as a priority, they may be included in local authorities' policies.

Policy officers were asked whether their authorities had written equal opportunities policies covering services to children, whether these had been implemented, and whether they undertook any ethnic monitoring of day care workers or children attending day care services. In addition they were asked whether the section 19 Review had been translated into any other languages besides English. This was an area where written policy did not necessarily reflect practice, so the absence of a policy did not always mean nothing was happening. Similarly, the existence of a policy in itself did not guarantee changes in practice. Nevertheless, eleven authorities had an equal opportunities policy, eight of which reported making some progress towards its implementation. Half of these eight were enabler authorities. One indicator of progress was collecting information on the ethnic backgrounds of workers in their own and independent services. Eleven authorities were doing this in some or all of the services available, usually in local authority services; and eight authorities were collecting similar information on the children attending services. No authorities had translated the section 19 Review into any languages besides English. Table 2.4 summarises progress in this field.

**Table 2.4: Summary of progress in the area of equal opportunities policies and implementation for day care services**

| Equal Opportunities policy N = 17 | Work on policy implementation | Ethnic monitoring of day care workers | Ethnic monitoring of children in day care services | Section 19 Review translated into any other languages |
|---|---|---|---|---|
| 11 | 8 | 11 (some or all services covered) | 8 (some or all services covered) | 0 |

There was no clear association between policy types and reported progress in this area beyond a tendency for enabler authorities to take a broader remit of 'equal opportunities' into consideration. However, it did appear from the comments of policy officers that the Children Act and

Guidance had helped give attention to the issue of equal opportunities. Some specific examples of changes in practice in individual local authorities, as a result of or in tandem with the Act, included:

- Anti-bias training group: a multi-disciplinary group making training available as part of a county wide training strategy.
- Complaints procedure: the Children Act led procedure has a panel that includes representatives chosen to reflect the ethnic composition of the local population.
- Training strategy: all senior managers with responsibility for service provision undertake awareness training; the practice and procedure guide has been revised.

Local authorities were at strikingly different stages in their inclusion of equal opportunities within policies. In some areas, the attention given to equal opportunities in the Children Act had led to policies being developed for the first time. One respondent (from a minimalist authority) said that 'for us [there has been] an impact because the fact that it was in legislation has enabled us to mention it in draft policy documents'. In another (an enabler provider) authority, the Children Act had no, or very little impact because equal opportunities 'were pretty well advanced...diversity issues were never mentioned with reference to the Children Act'.

Monitoring the ethnic background of day care workers and the usage of day care services posed some problems. In one local authority there was some resistance to the idea of ethnic monitoring based on categories of 'ethnic origin'; 'preferred language' was used instead. Several local authorities found it easier to monitor their own services than services in the independent sector, although one local authority used its information service to monitor all day care workers within each establishment when they registered for inclusion in the information service. Monitoring usage by children tended to be better established within education services, followed by local authority day nurseries.

In some areas there had been discussion about whether minority ethnic groups constituted a priority group for services. One policy officer pointed out that a policy switch away from identification of children 'in need' based on groups and towards individuals had had the effect of losing a focus on minority ethnic groups, but a greater attention was paid to each individual child's race, religion and culture. In another authority which contained areas with large minority ethnic populations, some problems arose in catering for the sometimes conflicting needs of *each* discrete group, sometimes within the same services.

*Voluntary organisations and ethnic diversity*

The service providers survey indicated that while about half of day care services have minority ethnic children, fewer services employ minority ethnic staff (Moss et al., 1995, tables 1 and 2). Voluntary organisations raised a number of issues in response to a question about the way local authorities handled 'equal opportunities and issues of ethnic diversity'. Firstly, several respondents noted that there is an 'attitudinal' problem within day care services. Some of the comments were:

> *People are frightened of it.*
>
> *I'm glad they don't push it too hard with childminders as it would put them off. Needs a very softly, softly approach.*
>
> *The local authority is willing to go along with it but there's a lot of lip service at grass roots level.*

A common theme here is the perception that issues of ethnic diversity are relevant only where there is a sizeable minority ethnic population, often expressed crudely as 'we don't have black children round here'.

A second and related problem is that of encouraging 'black' and Asian parents to use day care services. Mention was made above of a preference for facilities where children can speak their own language. A representative of a private day nurseries association voiced some possible reasons for a lack of take up:

> *the only reason given is [that they use the] extended family, or they are unemployed. For us Asian children are middle class and educated. There is fear and a lack of understanding. A lot of schools with Asian children have a nursery unit.*

A third problem is that most day care workers are 'white'. In some areas there had been specific attempts to encourage 'black' and Asian women to work in day care. One childminding representative said that through such a project she saw 'what kinds of problems they would have as minders ...they suffered a lot of abuse, say in parks, because they preferred to mind Asian children'.

Another respondent pointed out that such projects needed co-operation between the advice agencies and the local authority to ensure that they have the confidence of the community. She continued:

> *one project was set up in an area where 75 per cent are Asian, but can't get the involvement of Asian families. They can't get the co-operation of the agencies to make the project work.*

Many voluntary sector respondents argued that education and training were a vital key to improving the way in which issues of ethnic diversity were handled in day care services. This included training for day care officers as well as providers. While some said there was a resistance to training, others said this could be overcome by integrating equal opportunities training within other subjects. Two respondents gave examples of how training was being delivered in their areas:

- For playgroup leaders: five hours awareness course, plus a twenty-hour course covering a wider spectrum such as disability, race, culture and sexuality.
- An anti-bias training group where all organisations are represented sets up training days to look at positive images, resources, ways of ensuring children are involved and understand.

Finally, one respondent referred to the high proportion of ethnic minorities living in the area and said

> *we just got on with it. It had a high profile at one point, but it's just the norm around here.*

Promoting equal opportunities awareness within all day care services and encouraging access to, and confidence in, services for minority ethnic parents were at widely varying points among this sample of local authorities. The Children Act has succeeded in making the issue a 'live' one, although one by no means universally accepted as relevant or appropriate to all day care providers.

*Promoting provision for all children*

The main method of expansion of publicly-funded services for young children during the implementation period was the promotion of nursery education. Between 1991 and 1994, there was an 8 per cent increase in places for three and four year-olds in nursery classes and schools in the sample local authorities.

Some local authorities in the sample were able to promote general services for young children by combining various sources of funding. These included nursery education funded by the local education authority; funding for out-of-school care by TECs; child care elements of City Challenge bids; and grants to subsidise playgroup fees and training for playgroup workers and childminders. Some of these sources had conditions attached; our attention was drawn to one in particular – the TEC funding for out-of-school services required the services to be self funding within one year of operation which often limited the likely beneficiaries of the service to those children whose parents could afford to pay, and not those children living in areas of social disadvantage. Some examples of local authority initiatives to promote services for all children since the Children Act are shown in box 2.3.

**Box 2.3**

**Examples of local authority initiatives to promote services for all children**

- Grant aid to playgroups: £93,000 over 6 years in one local authority.
- Training support for playgroups: linking 70 infant schools with playgroups to provide teacher support in playgroups.
- Training and support to childminders: £60,000 in one local authority.
- Development officers: to provide support to groups, information to parents and develop services.
- Jointly funded posts: by TEC and social services department for out of school development officer; and by Taskforce and social service department for full day care development officer.
- Conversion of surplus school accommodation to nursery classes.
- Community business scheme: for childminders and schools to offer 'wrap around care'.

**Evaluation of the Act**

At the time of implementation of the Children Act, local authorities were at widely varying starting points in terms of the level of day care and educational provision for children under five, the political commitment to such provision, and dedicated policy officer time and resources to progress duties and powers under the new legislation. These differences in starting points tended to determine the view each local authority adopted concerning the significance of the Act, and can still be seen three years after implementation. Some local authorities have seen the Act as confirmation of their existing policies and practice, some have seen the Act as posing opportunities for exploring new means of delivering services, and others have seen the Act as requiring modest changes to the way they provide 'family support' services. In other words there was a tendency for local authorities and their policy officers to interpret the Act's duties and powers in the light of existing local policies and practice.

This chapter has highlighted differences in local authorities' methods of implementing the Act by focusing on traditionalist, enabling and minimalist styles found in the sample of local authorities. Progress with some aspects of implementation, such as monitoring and information services, were not clearly associated with these groupings, but one feature of provision within the enabling authorities requires specific mention. Among the enabling authorities there tended to be a culture of commitment not just to the age group, but also to extending access to all children, regardless of parental means, disability or 'race'. These authorities were prepared to do this by imaginative means, working across traditional divides and with all constituencies interested in early years.

One influence at a national level is the tradition of a residual public provision of day care places. Beyond the duty to provide a family centre in each local authority, the Children Act did not set out to increase the supply of publicly-funded places. Rather, it focused on formalising the process of gaining access to publicly-funded places, by introducing the term 'in need', and by emphasising the 'family support' role of public day care. The evidence at a local level suggests the emphasis on family support and children in need has been largely uncontroversial. The principle that children 'in need' require day care facilities was and is well accepted. The problems that were drawn to the research team's attention were the means of delivering day care services from within a system of 'sponsorship' that relies on the private and voluntary sector. Evidence from the service providers survey (Moss et al., 1995) and from the comments of voluntary sector representatives suggested that day care providers in the independent sector are very willing to do the work, but without proper advisory support, training and equipment, the facilities can feel under intense pressure. It is possible, or even likely, that children 'in need' are being served by a very under-resourced independent sector.

For children with disabilities, brought into the mainstream of social service provision for the first time, the Children Act held a promise of more, and better co-ordinated, services. The evidence here was of a perception of marked improvement on the part of the policy officers, some of whom were new to the area of delivering these services, and more mixed views on the part of the voluntary sector.

Perhaps the most significant change to the overall picture for early years provision is the supply in nursery education. The renewed national interest in nursery education has been felt in local authorities during the course of the study. Changes of political complexion in four of the sample local authorities following local government elections in 1993 and 1994 led three of them to declare an interest in expanding nursery education. One county council had already agreed considerable extra resources to this effect.

Turning to the local influences on policy, a recurrent theme was the prevalence of budget cuts. Reference has been made earlier to the problem of inadequate information about financial resources in local authorities. The perception of policy officers was of an increase in resources for early years but one constantly moderated by budget cuts in both services and in policy officer time. In five authorities, it was clear that budget constraints were having major consequences for the organisation and delivery of services. While one had managed to forestall likely substantial cuts to services for young children by creating a discrete early years unit under the education department, in the other four cases budget cuts were having a generally detrimental effect on the level of services and policy resources for the development of services. In one case the entire policy process had come to a standstill because of 'frozen' posts.

One local authority faced *both* budget cuts and changes in political direction at the final phase of the fieldwork. Severe financial difficulties for the authority meant officers were being asked to cut and juggle resources, with no policy direction to help establish priorities. This, combined with a general absence of clear policy making within the authority, was reported to have left policy officers very unclear about the direction to pursue. They felt pulled in opposing directions.

The final point concerns the indigenous culture and context for the provision of services for young children. While local differences have always existed in the commitment to services for young children, in three cases it appeared that local factors were more significant in shaping the direction of policy than the Children Act. These tended to be authorities which already had an established corporate/joint policy making process, ones which had recently undertaken widespread consultation and implementation of the consequent recommendations, and ones where the strength, commitment and participation of the voluntary sector were given a high priority by the responsible council committee structure.

**Lessons from the Research**

- Services such as family centres can successfully be developed in 'partnership' with the voluntary sector.
- Promoting the use of private and voluntary sector day care services is a useful method of expansion of day care for children in need.
- Sponsorship budgets require both careful monitoring of usage and local control over spending to offer the widest possible access to services.
- Day care providers need support and training to enable them to offer an appropriate service to children 'in need'.
- For children with disabilities, local authority partnership with the voluntary sector is necessary to make use of this sector's expertise in the field.
- Every effort should be made to work across departments and agencies to avoid voluntary organisations (and children and families) being caught between conflicting policies.
- A local authority-wide 'one stop' information service for parents offers considerable benefits.
- A sustained and high level commitment to the principles and practice of equal opportunities is necessary to make the ethos of the Act a reality.

CHAPTER

# 3 Co-ordination of Services for Young Children

**Mano Candappa**

## Background

Under section 19 of the Children Act, social services departments and local education authorities have a duty jointly to conduct and publish a report on a Review of day care services for children under eight in their area at least once every three years. Although the legislation 'does not require the two authorities to review nursery and primary education facilities as such...they are required to inform themselves about quantity and availability' (DoH, 1991: para. 9.6). In elaborating on local authorities' oversight and co-ordination function under the Act, the Guidance recommends a co-ordinated approach to day care and education services as 'a means of ensuring that all children...have access to a good quality curriculum or programme with continuity of experience and smooth transition to other forms of day care or education' (DoH, 1991: para. 1.16). Co-ordination is required at three levels:

- policy making;
- day-to-day operation of services;
- between staff working in different settings.

The model envisaged is of separate day care and education systems, working together across separate operational frameworks. The Guidance stresses the need for local authorities also to 'have regard to' links with other departments and other statutory authorities, such as health authorities and NHS Trusts, and with local voluntary organisations, community groups, minority ethnic interests, the private childcare sector, and employer interests in planning and developing services.

Patterns and trends in services for young children reveal a need for co-ordination of services. Some of the main characteristics of services as summarised by Pugh (1992a) include:

- services based on different underpinning ideologies, having different aims and purposes;

- unco-ordinated services run by different local authority departments, by health authorities, voluntary agencies, community groups, private individuals and companies, and employers;
- uneven distribution of services across the country;
- low levels of public funding of services;
- a growing reliance on the independent sector in service development.

In short, the general picture is of a fragmented collection of services with little overall planning.

The main local authority providing departments – social services, education, and leisure services – by and large do not have a history of consultation or joint working in services for young children; even though joint working between education and social services has been encouraged since the early part of the century, and more recently advocated in circulars LASSL (76)5, and LASSL (78)1. Indeed, the care – education – play divide which these departments represent, is often characterised by jealously-guarded professional boundaries, different ideologies and priorities, and different traditions and patterns of working.

**The Wider Debate**

In discussing the local authority's co-ordination function, the Guidance points out that the Act cannot succeed 'without effective inter-departmental collaboration at all levels' (DoH, 1991, para. 1.8). The Guidance also speaks of duties and powers relating to co-operation between departments under the Act (ibid., para. 1.13); and in various places it refers to *co-ordination, co-operation* and *collaboration*. However neither the Guidance nor the Act clarify the meanings of, or the distinctions between, the respective terms. This is hardly surprising because, as Hallett and Birchall's (1992) literature review suggests, there is some ambiguity in the meaning of these terms. They have been used variously by different authors, with some using 'common-sense' definitions, others proposing their own, and still others using the terms 'co-ordination' and 'collaboration' synonymously. Authors such as Challis et al. (1988) point to the rhetorical function served by the very ambiguity of the word 'co-ordination'.

A useful definition is offered by Bond et al. (1985), in which 'collaboration' is used as a blanket term that covers different patterns of joint working between individuals or groups within an organisation. Taken in this sense, collaboration can be distinguished from co-operation and co-ordination, terms which Mulford and Rogers (1982) use to describe specific ways of inter-organisational working: 'co-operation' involves individual organisations' goals and objectives and no formal rules, whilst 'co-ordination' involves formal rules and joint goals and activities. 'Co-ordination' therefore poses more of a threat to autonomy than does 'co-operation'. Used in this sense, local authority departments such as social services and education which operate in a fairly autonomous way, can be considered as separate organisations in terms of working relationships. Thus informal contact and working to separate goals can be referred to as co-operation, and formally structured working relationships with jointly agreed goals as co-ordination. By this definition, 'co-ordination' can also be used to refer to structured working relationships between local authorities and outside bodies (such as health authorities and voluntary sector organisations), and co-operation for more informal working. Collaboration on the other hand, following Bond et al., would refer to working relationships between different units within single departments.

Akin to the terms co-operation, co-ordination, and collaboration in social policy and relevant to the subject of services for young children are the terms *corporate policy* and *integrated service*, both of which are referred to in the Guidance. Thus a local authority as a corporate body may agree an early years policy which requires co-ordinated or co-operative working across many different departments. A contrasting approach would be where an authority has integrated all services for young children within a single department, and where collaboration between different units in that department may be envisaged in policy implementation.

Co-ordination has three different aspects, and can as such be considered: in terms of organisational arrangements; as a process; and in terms of its outputs (Challis et al., 1988). In the literature is the idea that through co-ordinated working agencies can achieve something more than 'the sum of their parts', i.e. objectives that were unreachable or difficult to achieve on their own, or by other ways of co-operative working. Indeed, this idea is apparent in the Guidance, where a co-ordinated approach is seen as a means of ensuring the quality and accessibility of services for young children. But conversely, as Hallett and Birchall (1992) point out, 'co-operation and consensus are not necessary and inevitable components of co-ordination' (ibid.: 12).

The different dimensions involved in attempting to co-ordinate a service need also to be considered. To quote Hallett and Birchall (1992):

> *It is frequently the case that policy objectives are equivocal, multiple and possibly conflicting, as are organisational goals...Often, however, policy objectives are not spelled out...Even when objectives are clearly defined and articulated by politicians and civil servants at the top of the policy process, others in the system may perceive them differently. Notably, this includes those with responsibilities for implementation, who interpret and remake policy as they carry it out...Within the ranks of the policy implementers, too, there are likely to be differences of view between for example, those at the top and the bottom of welfare hierarchies ...Yet other perspectives may be offered by users of services (ibid.: 15).*

Co-ordinating a service, therefore, involves more than setting up structures and communicating information; policy is subject to mediation by implementing actors, with their individual value bases. Other mediating factors also come into play: for example, environmental factors, and particularly in the context of this study, competing legislation and budgetary considerations, which cannot just be 'co-ordinated away'.

There is also a distinction between voluntary co-ordination – where agencies choose to engage in co-ordination, and mandated co-ordination – the situation as under the Children Act, where they are required by law to establish inter-organisational linkages. When organisations choose to work together it is usually for perceived mutual benefit and, if it is to be successful, would among other things involve a positive attitude towards and a recognised need for co-ordination (Whetten, 1981). In mandated co-ordination, the overriding factor is awareness of the mandate, and the key problem for implementers then becomes how to secure adherence to the mandate. Here, some useful suggestions may be taken from the study by Bradley (1982) where identified factors for successful co-ordination include:

- clarity and simplicity of arrangements and procedures;
- a need for communication, consultation, negotiation;
- mutual awareness, respect and support between all groups and sectors involved.

Similarly Pugh (1992b) suggests that in services for young children effective co-ordination requires, *inter alia*, a clear policy and development plan, a supporting committee and administrative structure, and clear support from elected members and chief officers.

Debate about co-ordination over the past two decades has focused on the need to make better use of resources and to provide a more flexible and responsive service to children and their parents. A number of reports have called for a better co-ordinated and more coherent national policy, notably the Rumbold Committee (DES, 1990), the Equal Opportunities Commission (1990), the Association of Metropolitan Authorities (AMA) (1991), the National Consumer Council (1991), the National Commission on Education (1993), and the Royal Society of Arts (Ball, 1994). The AMA report, whilst recommending that children's services should be integrated within one department, did not see co-ordination within existing frameworks as a 'viable option'; but stated however that establishing a new children's department was 'perhaps a bridge too far at this stage' (ibid., p.48). More recently, a National Children's Bureau study (McQuail and Pugh, 1995) drew attention to the relationship between the aims of a service and its supporting organisational structures.

In the sections that follow, efforts at joint working in the study authorities in relation to policy planning and the section 19 Review will be considered in terms of structures, of process, and of outcomes, using mini-case studies as illustration. The development and implementation of children 'in need' policies will not be discussed, since this has been the subject of another study for the Department of Health, and co-ordinated working in this area has been covered in that study (see Aldgate et al., 1994).

## Implementation Three Years after the Act

*Models of service development*

In the light of the above discussion, a number of different conceptual models along which policy on services for young children is developed and delivered can be envisaged. A first model is of authorities with all services for young children integrated into one department. At present, authorities with such integrated departments are more likely to be those with a heavy investment in services, and as the major service providers they place less reliance on the independent sector in developing services. In such a model the voluntary and private sectors could have minimal inputs into policy development; these can thus also be considered as the more *controlling* authorities.

A second model is that of the more *enabling* authority, where there is a greater reliance on the independent sector for provision of services. Within this model policy and services are developed through co-ordinated working with the independent sector and other statutory bodies; or through co-operative working with these agencies. In the first case, working arrangements would be characterised by formal structures and shared goals, while in the second there would be few formal rules or jointly agreed goals.

A third model encompasses those authorities that adopt a *laissez-faire* approach, where service development is left up to the vagaries of the market, with a minimalist role for the local authority, and where co-ordination could be seen to be of less importance.

The above, it must be stressed, are relatively 'pure' types. In practice, elements of each can be found in the other models. For example, an authority with an integrated department might work co-operatively or in consultation with the independent sector and other statutory bodies; and a laissez-faire authority might similarly consult or work co-operatively with other agencies. So too, an authority might combine some co-ordinated working with co-operative working on other issues. The models are, however, a useful aid to analysis.

*Types of co-ordinating structure*

Working within the broad parameters of the above models, a typology of co-ordinating mechanisms in the study authorities has been developed, to reflect existing structures, rather than the 'pure' types. In this, an authority's relationship with the independent sector has been taken as a key dimension. Thus, authorities that did not involve the voluntary and private sectors in service planning are described as *controlling* if they were also high providers of services themselves. Authorities that involved the independent sector, either directly or indirectly (through consultation) in the planning of service development are described as *enabling/consultative*. Those authorities with low levels of own provision that did not work with the independent sector in service development are treated as being within the *laissez-faire* model, even if they had structured working relations within the statutory sector. At one end of the continuum, therefore, are the high service providers: the *integrated* authorities; the *co-ordinated/controlling* authorities (with structured working relations across the statutory sector only); and *other controlling* authorities (with no co-ordinated working even across local authority departments). In the middle are the *enabling/consultative* authorities. At the other end are the low providers: the *other co-ordinated* authorities being those with structured working relations within the statutory sector, while the 'pure' *laissez-faire* authorities did not engage in co-ordinated working. The development of co-ordinating structures along these lines over the study period is as seen in table 3.1.

**Table 3.1: Development of co-ordinating structures from Stage 1 to Stage 3**

| Co-ordinating Structures | | | | | | |
|---|---|---|---|---|---|---|
| Stage | Integrated | Co-ordinated/ controlling | Other controlling | Enabling/ consultative | Other co-ordinated | *Laissez-faire* |
| 1992/3 (n = 18) | 1 | 3 | – | 7 | 2 | 5 |
| 1994/5 (n = 17) | 3 | – | 1 | 10 | 3 | – |

It will be seen that three of the 17 authorities had integrated early years departments by the final stage of the study – representing an overall movement towards integration by two authorities since the first stage. But none of these represented a totally controlling model: one of them had co-opted a representative of a body co-ordinating voluntary sector activity on its Early Years Sub-Committee; another included a voluntary sector representative on a consultative group set up to advise its new integrated service; and the third had an under eights liaison committee for advice/consultation, which included local interests on its membership. But since in all cases the local authority was the main provider of services, they will be considered within the controlling model.

One authority that was described as co-ordinated/controlling at the first stage had no operating co-ordinating structures for the development of services for young children at the second stage. An authority which provides 'play care', and extended day care in conjunction with nursery education in addition to its eight day nurseries, it had moved all its provision for children aged under eight, with the exception of its day nurseries (which remained in social services) to its education department. Its relationship with the independent sector remained unchanged, i.e., the voluntary sector was generously supported through grant-aiding, but no independent sector representatives were involved in the authority's planning processes. While this authority cannot therefore be placed among the 'integrated' authorities, it still remains within the 'controlling' model.

Ten of the remaining 13 authorities were within the 'enabling' model. They all demonstrate joint working in policy development with other statutory and independent sector agencies, which includes the use of some formal co-ordinating structures. This represents a movement of four authorities from the broad *laissez-faire* category to the enabling/consultative model over the period of the study. Authorities whose forums were merely for information sharing/gathering are not included in this model.

No authorities conformed to the pure *laissez-faire* model by the final stage. However, three authorities who had developed structured working relations among local authority departments and with other statutory agencies, but did not consult with the independent sector in service planning, are included as 'other co-ordinate' within the broad *laissez-faire* model.

Co-ordinating mechanisms in place range from (i) those at local authority-level only (such as joint sub-committees at the political level, and inter-departmental working groups at officer level); to (ii) those involving the local authority and other statutory agencies (such as health authorities); through to (iii) those that include local authority members and/or officers, with representatives from other statutory agencies, independent providers, community organisations and users. Typically, structures demonstrating the greatest breadth were those Under Eights sub-committees, and those forums which sought representation from all sectors. Equally, there were structures that did not include either the political and/or the community and user ends of the spectrum.

Most authorities had some co-ordinated working with other local authority departments; and the majority of authorities also had structured working relations with health authorities, though these were not confined to day care services, and some pre-dated the implementation of the Children Act. A small number of authorities additionally had a corporate or joint-funded early years post. Overall, this represents a continued growth in co-ordinating mechanisms over the first three years of the implementation of the Children Act.

The main mechanism used for formal contact with the voluntary and private sectors by local authorities were forums (sometimes described as liaison committees). At the first stage of this study, forums/liaison committees operated at local authority-level in ten authorities, with some having local feeder forums, while in some others forums operated at local level only. The majority of these had been initiated by the local authority. At the second stage, the overall number of authority-wide forums had increased to 12, with two of the original ten given an expanded role. In one other of the original number, an authority-wide discussion forum was replaced by a more comprehensive system of local forums. This authority had also used a forum-type consultative group to advise its new integrated service.

In three authorities there was no forum-type mechanism, even just at local level. In terms of the typologies discussed earlier, of these authorities two were more controlling authorities with high levels of own provision; the other was a county with low levels of own provision and a *laissez-faire* approach to service development. Predictably, the growth of forums was concentrated among the enabling authorities.

These various co-ordinating structures and models present specific problems or raise issues on which the discussion will now centre. In particular, co-ordinating or integrating services for young children involves working across professional boundaries which need to be surmounted to achieve effective functioning of the system; various co-ordinating structures, including forum models, carry different political and other implications; these structures and patterns of working can have implications for the manner in which the section 19 Review is carried out. The rest of this chapter will consider these issues, focusing in on 'critical cases' from the fieldwork.

*Overcoming professional boundaries*

Developing a corporate early years policy, a measure suggested in the Guidance (para. 4.4) is likely to bring into relief the tensions inherent in the care–education–play divide mentioned near the beginning of this chapter. For its success, officers from participating departments need to cross the conceptual boundaries of their departmental thinking, their traditions, and older ways of planning. Some of these dimensions are exemplified in the cases of two local authorities, referred to as Authorities A and B.

In Authority A, a large northern county, the first section 19 Review had highlighted the need for a corporate policy. An Early Years Policy Group was formed, incorporating members from the Review steering group (which comprised officers from the social services and education departments), and the process of agreeing the policy spanned the work of both groups. The process is described by an officer who served on both these groups:

> *we were all strangers – never even met socially. We started a long way back, getting together to share ideas before we could do the Review...to do that, we had to find a common language...*

Through this long drawn-out process the policy was developed, incorporating guiding principles, each with objectives, strategy and targets. The targets exemplify the intention of co-ordinated and co-operative working to a great extent, with the social services and education departments taking joint lead responsibility for the implementation of many targets. For other targets, one or other department takes lead responsibility for implementation.

In Authority B the first Review and corporate early years policy developed more or less in tandem, and the experience was more fraught, by comparison. In this London borough, initial discussions within their first Children Act Review Group (which included an officer from a central policy unit in addition to officers from the three main providing departments) had suggested the need for co-ordinating services for young children. This resulted in the formation of an Early Years Strategy Group. The group took nearly two years to develop an agreed Early Years Strategy, which 'sought to overcome the traditional care-education-play divide', and contained a three-year action plan, into which the Review's programme of action dovetailed. The corporate strategy contrasts with the tradition of separate departmental policies developed in parallel, with limited co-operative working between some key officers within them, which preceded it.

The process of arriving at that document was described as 'torture at various points' by a member of the group, due to competing philosophies and departmental rivalries among members. It seemed clear that without the vital role played by the central policy unit in co-ordinating the group's work, arriving at a strategy would have proved a much more difficult, if not impossible task.

The experience of both authorities underlines the point made above of the need for early years professionals to move beyond their traditional boundaries to an appreciation of the complementary roles each plays in a child's development, and the difficulties this presents. These difficulties could similarly affect the working of an integrated young children's department, as discussed below.

Of the three integrated authorities in our sample, one in particular exemplifies how persistent professional boundaries can be, and how this can affect the successful running of an integrated early years service. Authority C is a northern metropolitan borough. At the first stage of the research, it was reported that a proposal to locate young children's services within education was before Committee. A phased transfer was envisaged, and the first section 19 Review was used as the starting point for the new service.

By the third stage, an Integrated Young Children's Service had been formed, with the entire service managed by education. But, in the words of a senior officer, the 'initial welcome had been replaced by divisions based on the old services'. She commented that the 'language of the discourse was a significant issue...We desperately need a new language to express a new service'.

The experiences of each of the three authorities discussed above demonstrates some of the difficulties inherent in attempting to make very different agencies work together. But more than that, it reinforces the point made earlier about the difference between making policy and implementing it: that officials make and re-make policy as they carry it out. On a practical level it points to the urgent need for finding a 'common language' in bridging the care–education–play divide.

*Co-ordinating structures: inclusive and exclusive models*

Co-ordinating structures developed by local authorities typically comprised one or more of joint committees, sub-committees, or member panels at the *political level*; corporate groups or inter-agency groups for service planning at *officer level*; and forums or liaison committees at *grass-roots level*. Examples of the inclusive model (embracing all three levels) were found in seven authorities, while a further three were in the process of establishing such a model. Examples of the *exclusive* model (operating at just one or two levels) were found in the remaining seven authorities. Authorities A and D offer illustrations of the two models.

Authority A offers an example of an inclusive model. Here a pyramid of structures has been developed specific to services for young children, to which other co-ordinating structures are linked. At the top of the pyramid is an Early Years Sub-Committee, which is a joint sub-committee of the Social Services and Education Committees. This body includes co-opted representatives from outside organisations such as the PLA, the local branch of the NCMA, and a private day nurseries association. Co-opted members have a voice in debates, but no voting rights; and the Sub-Committee has advisory rather than policy-making status. But since its membership includes the chairs of both its parent committees, the distinction is academic.

At the next level is a County Early Years Forum, which acts as a consultative body to the Early Years Sub-Committee. The forum has an upper limit of 25 to its membership, which includes an elected Member from the Sub-Committee, and representatives of service providers and users, and which is open to annual review.

The bottom level of the pyramidal structure is in the early stages of development, and when complete will consist of local forums which will feed into the County Forum. Once a network of such forums has been established, the three tiers of local and county forums and sub-committee together are expected to provide an effective framework for co-ordination, consultation and policy development.

Linked to, but not part of the pyramidal structure, is a Review Steering Group. An officer group drawn from all departments providing services for young children, it is linked to the 'pyramid' through its membership, many of whom are involved with the forums, and through the Sub-Committee, to which it reports and is responsible. Figure 3.1 shows the levels and composition of the different groups, and how they relate to each other.

Authority D is an outer London borough where co-ordinating structures are less inclusive than in Authority A. Here, prior to the Children Act there was little co-ordinated or co-operative working between departments or with the voluntary sector. With the Act an Under Eights Coordinator was appointed by the education department. Soon after, she set up a forum of people with an interest in early years, but which was not intended to feed directly into any local authority process. The Act also provided the impetus for setting up a Disability Register Working Group, which included strong representation from a parents' group. Since then there has been a growth in joint working, more particularly with the setting up of a Children's Services Planning Group, with representatives from social services, education, leisure services, housing, health, and the local council for voluntary services. Most recently an Under Eights Corporate Group has been formed comprising representatives from local authority departments, and it is hoped to enlarge membership to include health and the voluntary sector – thus taking on some of the characteristics usually associated with forums (see Early Years Forums below).

One of the main recommendations of the Children's Services Planning Group is expected to be around methods of joint working. A children's services planning day which the group had organised showed that there

**Figure 3.1: Co-ordinating structures Inclusive model**

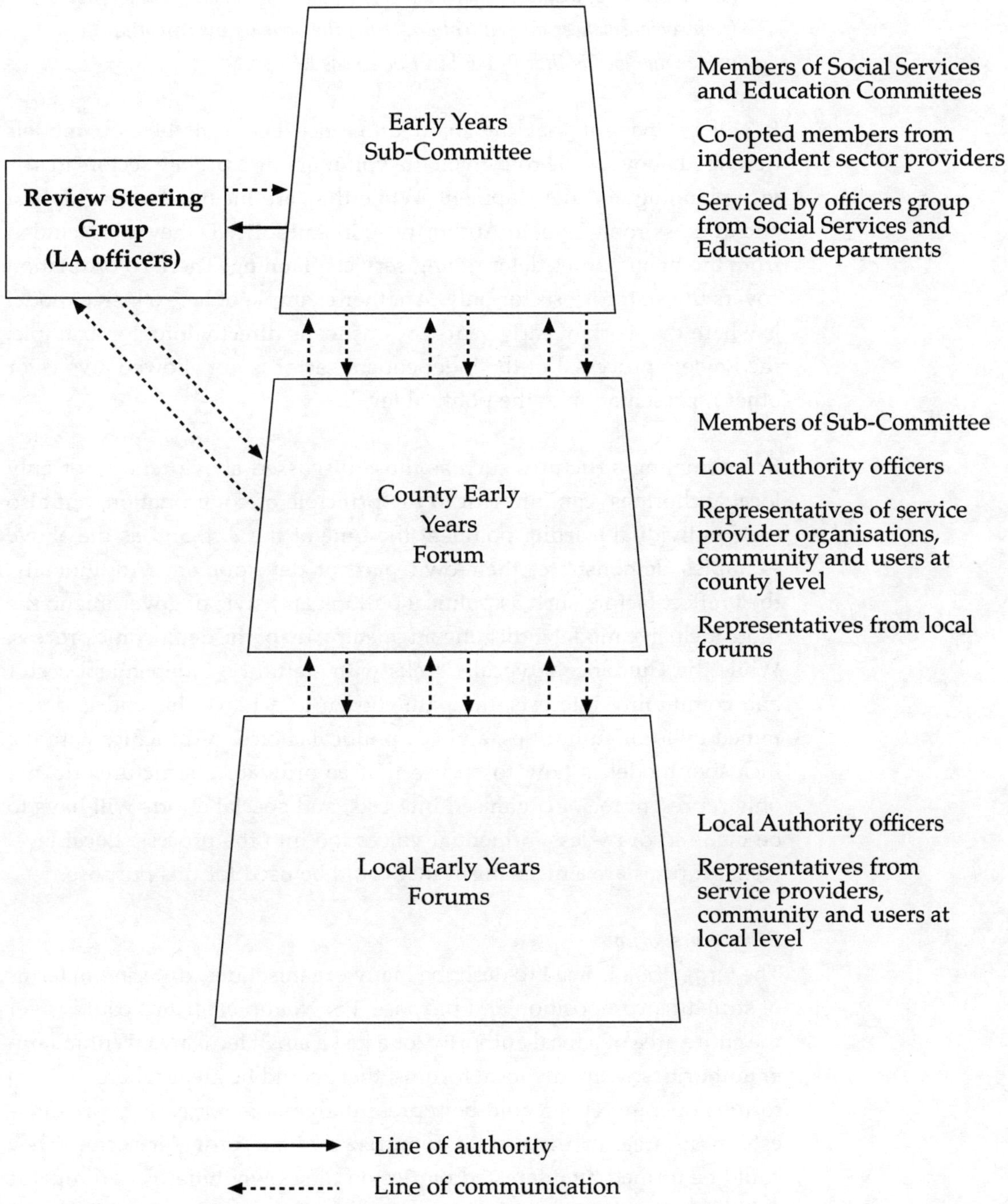

was also considerable parental support for this. But it was becoming clear that the authority's co-ordinating structures were insufficient for its objectives. A senior officer commented:

> *One of the problems is the committee structure. One suggestion from [social services] members is to have a joint panel of members and officers from social services and education. [But] the view of one education committee member is that it wouldn't be so easy.*

It will be evident that the main difference between the two models described above is the role given the voluntary and private sectors in service planning and development. While they are included at the highest and at grass-roots level in Authority A, in Authority D they are excluded from the main bodies determining service planning. There co-ordination covers the statutory sector only. Another example of an exclusive model is where the work of early years forums feeds directly into, for example, the Review process, but the independent sector is not allowed a voice or other representation at the political level.

Co-ordinating structures such as those discussed above reflect not only local authorities' commitment to the principle of co-ordination, but also their individual starting points at the time of the Act, and as the above examples demonstrate, their own pace of development. Additionally, they reflect factors such as political outlook and style of government: the more inclusive model indicating an opening up of the democratic process. While the Guidance advocates links with statutory, independent sector and community interests, the path chosen to achieve this end is determined by local authorities, and is a political choice. A difficulty with the inclusive model is how to ensure that co-ordinating structures do not only represent major organised interests, and special efforts will have to be made to draw less influential voices too into the process. Local level feeder forums are a mechanism that could be used for this purpose.

*Early years forums*

The term *forum* is used to describe many organisations, differing in terms of structure, composition and purpose. For example, forums could cover the entire area of a local authority, or a just a small local area. Within larger authorities with only local forums, there could be areas where no local forums operate. They could be representative of major early years interests in an area, or they could comprise a single provider sector. They could be formed by interested parties on their own initiative, or impetus could be provided from the local authority. They could operate for information sharing, as a pressure group or more directly as part of an authority's policy development mechanism. And so on. The definition of 'forum' used in this study extends only to those representing voluntary sector interests among others, and carrying an authority-wide brief.

A model favoured by the National Early Years Network (NEYN, formerly VOLCUF) is that of a body that seeks to represent the interests of children in their early years, to which every individual parent/carer and every service user or provider can make representations. The forum must involve the voluntary sector, and to be most effective must be independent of the local authority. The forum could, amongst other things, coordinate and liaise between services, have a consultative role in the development of services, be a focus for collecting information, as well as lobby and have an advocacy role (VOLCUF, undated). The need for securing adequate resources for the forum is recognised, and seeking support from the local authority for this purpose is suggested (Ball and Stone, 1991).

In the authorities in this study, such a model was not found in its 'pure' form. One resembling it in structure is that developed in Authority A, as described earlier. But here the impetus is provided by the local authority, which is responsible for organising and running the forum system. Its purpose therefore does not correspond to that in the NEYN model. In Authority A the forum forms an integral part of early years policy development, and can be seen as a widening of the democratic process and a move towards empowering of childcare interests by the authority.

A contrasting model is provided by Authority D. While the local education authority's Under Eights Co-ordinator was responsible for setting it up and takes an active part in its operation, it is intended to be a grassroots organisation only, and functions without the involvement of the hierarchy in the authority. Its objectives are also limited: it is a forum for sharing ideas and expertise in meeting the needs of children aged under eight in the borough. Thus while it performs a function in bringing together people with an interest in children aged under eight in the authority, it does not and is not intended to directly influence local authority early years policy planning.

Twelve authorities reported authority-wide forums in their area, and broadly speaking, two models of forum emerged in terms of purpose, as illustrated above. A forum with the narrower remit could be initiated equally by a local authority or by other interests, and of the 12 authorities three reported such a model. Two of these had been formed expressly without the involvement of social services departments, though both had support from the education authority but to different extents.

Forums whose remit involves contributing directly to policy development however, must necessarily be recognised, if not supported, by the local authority, whether through direct involvement and constitution, or through funding. In the latter case the authority will need to recognise the validity of the forum as a channel for consulting with wider interests, as suggested in the NEYN model. In this study, most of the authorities where forums formed part of the mechanism for policy development were the more enabling authorities, and also those whose co-ordinating structures extended from the political through to the independent sector; and it seems to mark a trend among local authorities to use forums in this way. But it must be pointed out that neither all enabling authorities nor all the more inclusive authorities subscribed to this model of forum.

A final point concerns the need for adequate funding for a forum, however limited its aims. This point was brought home most clearly in the case of Authority E, a large metropolitan council with both local and authority-wide forums which predated the Children Act. Its early years forum was formed to establish links between the statutory and voluntary sectors with the aim of promoting high standards of care, with the voluntary sector and education taking the lead in setting it up. The forum has an executive committee and is linked to local forums, which number over a dozen. The forum receives no funding but has been allowed the use of a limited amount of local education authority resources. To quote a member of its executive, the forum 'is carried on top of members' normal jobs'. Not having a funded worker has proved the forum's downfall: unable to function effectively the forum is splitting off into sectors representing different service provider interests, with each sector making its own funding arrangements. The forum vice-chair commented, 'splitting off was inevitable because of the funding...there's a limit to how long you can rely on everyone's goodwill'.

Authority E's experience can be contrasted with that of Authority D, whose forum had similar aims. There the forum continues to function with the voluntary sector and education taking the lead in its operation. The main difference is that in the case of Authority D, the Under Eights Coordinator's budget provides for its funding and support for activities it organises.

It seems clear from the above that securing funding must be a priority in setting up a forum. However, if as suggested by the NEYN the local authority is approached for funding, the terms of the funding should be negotiated so as to ensure that the remit and functioning of the forum is not compromised.

*The section 19 review*

The project period covered the completion of the first Reviews and preparations for the second. The first stage report outlined the various arrangements made by authorities for undertaking the first Reviews, and noted that the majority of Reviews were largely descriptive, with only about half the sample including any specific recommendations or action plans in them. The study undertaken by Elfer and McQuail (1996) for the Department of Health provides more detail and commentary on the first Reviews, while the Social Services Inspectorate (SSI, 1994) has provided a useful overview of them. This section considers the progress made on the second Reviews by the study authorities in terms of joint working and consultation as suggested in the Guidance, and in relation to the experience of the first Reviews.

Eleven of the 17 authorities in the study had begun work on the second Review at the time of the fieldwork. In all cases a group had been set up to steer the Review, and the emerging pattern is of two approaches to steering groups used in preparing the Review. Authority A is an example of the first approach. There, steering the Review is seen as the responsibility of the statutory sector, and the steering group comprises officers from local authority departments and a representative of the health authority. Members oversee the work of the group through regular reports to the Sub-Committee. Once a draft has been approved by Members it will be put out to wide consultation: a hundred copies are planned to be distributed, using the mechanism of the county and local forums for this purpose. Only one other authority subscribes to this model.

The remainder of the study authorities have taken the second approach. Here, conducting the Review is seen as a joint enterprise of the local authority and those representing day care interests within their area. This invariably includes the voluntary sector, and in fewer cases extends also to other service provider and community interests. Authority F, a large southern county, is an example of the latter group. Here the Review is led by officers from social services and education, assisted by a steering group composed of local authority officers, district councils, a health authority representative, representatives of all the major day care interests in the county, and a disability association. A Joint Member Panel oversees the work of the steering group. Once a consultation document has been prepared it is expected to be taken out to wide consultation using local forums (a county-level forum does not exist), parish councils, and so on for the purpose.

It will be observed that either of the above models could be used effectively in conducting the Review, since they reflect ownership of the Review rather than any other consideration. What is more important is how and to what extent non-statutory interests have been considered and consulted in reviewing services. There was no apparent relationship between local authority type and the organisation of the Review process – for example, of the two authorities in the first model, one was an integrated authority with high levels of its own provision, whilst the other was a more enabling and co-ordinated authority.

From the discussion on co-ordinating structures and forums above, it will be obvious that having broad representation on a Review steering group is not in itself sufficient to ensure that the concerns of all interested parties are given sufficient consideration, and indeed was not seen as such in any of the authorities subscribing to this model. What it allows, is an opportunity to tap into the experiences of a range of people in guiding the Review process before putting out to wider consultation. In the first model the same effects can be achieved through an on-going consultation with these interests, using the forum or similar mechanism; which again, is the process being followed in the two authorities in that model.

Work had not progressed very far on most of the Reviews at the time of the fieldwork, but in general the experience of the first Review had alerted authorities to its limitations, and the triennial Review was providing an opportunity to learn from it. Among the main lessons to emerge from the first Review was the need for greater and more systematic consultation, and for greater involvement of the voluntary sector. In particular the use of open meetings for consultation was found to be generally unsuccessful.

Data from stage three interviews with organisations representing independent sector providers suggest that their knowledge of and involvement in the first Reviews was indeed far from satisfactory. Of the 15 local NCMA representatives interviewed, four who had been in post at the time reported not having seen a copy of their authority's Review report.

Three of them did not expect to be involved in the second Review either. The level of knowledge of the Reviews by local PLA representatives was on the whole better, though one of them (based in a southern county) revealed that she did not know what the Review was. A range of comments made by representatives of independent sector providers on the Reviews are given in the box 3.1.

**Box 3.1**

**Comments on section 19 review by representatives of independent sector**

- '[The Review] was useful. We discussed it at the Under-8s Liaison Group... we were able to put things forward, to discuss, question anything'.(NCMA representative, northern county).
- 'I've seen a copy of the Review... I was very impressed with [the authority's] paperwork' (NCMA representative, London borough).
- 'We were not consulted initially, just had a token visit. The report was very, very basic...[The process is] much better this time round – they've taken on the broad criticisms' (NCMA representative, metropolitan borough).
- 'I was contacted over the first Review – it was token. The level of our involvement was unsatisfactory' (PLA representative, metropolitan borough).
- 'We had no inputs into the first Review; typical of this borough – always make up their mind and then tell us. That's their idea of consultation' (PLA representative, London borough).

The comments in box 3.1 illustrate both positive reactions and dissatisfaction with the Review process felt by some organisations, the last quoted particularly questioning the authority's model of consultation. As noted, most authorities were themselves less than satisfied with their consultation methods, and to better accomplish this at the second Review the majority of authorities had planned to use more formal mechanisms, such as the forum; although in the main the consultation process was largely unplanned at the time of the fieldwork.

One of the concerns of this study with regard to consultation, and one which emerged from the first stage of the study, is the involvement of minority ethnic communities in the Review process, as advocated in the Guidance. We noted that consultation with minority ethnic groups was not widespread, and where attempted was generally acknowledged to be unsuccessful. Similar concerns were voiced by Elfer and McQuail (1996). At this later stage of the study, we found the issue of consultation with minority ethnic interests to be a matter of concern for implementing officers, though again, the process of engaging in dialogue with them seemed unclear. Here, the literature on consulting with these groups suggests that consultation should be an ongoing process based on mutual respect; that there should be clarity about the purposes of consultation, with feedback provided on their outcomes (see Christie and Blunden, 1991; Dutt with St. Rose, undated; Gaster and Martin, 1993; Gill, 1985; Qaiyoom, 1992). Data from stage one of this study indicates that trust between a local authority and minority ethnic communities needs to be established before any meaningful consultation can take place. Evidence from the case studies suggests that largely untapped resources, such as a local education authority's intercultural support service, could have a knowledge, experience and contacts with minority ethnic communities that might usefully form the basis upon which trust could be built. Equally, a health authority's health visitor service could have a knowledge base and contacts which could prove similarly useful.

A last but most important issue concerns political support for the Review. Whilst carrying out the triennial Review of services is a statutory duty under the Children Act, its profile and scope will largely depend on the resources devoted to it, which in turn depends on the level of political support it receives. The study by Elfer and McQuail (1996) suggests, as do our first stage findings, that elected member involvement in the first Reviews was not at a desired level. Equally, many authorities acknowledged that their Reviews had been under-resourced, with officers hard pressed to carry out the Review in addition to their normal duties.

The second Reviews had not progressed sufficiently at the time of the fieldwork to allow us to comment on elected member involvement, but it was noted that at stage one of our study, members were involved on the steering groups of only two authorities. Member involvement in the Reviews of eight other authorities was reportedly through oversight and reporting to committee. It can be argued here that direct member involvement on steering groups, while being desirable, is not essential provided they are kept informed of their progress and difficulties being encountered, and members take an active interest in their work. Active member support for Review recommendations will however be essential for their resourcing and implementation.

*The co-ordination process: views from independent sector participants*

The difference between structure and process was noted earlier. The point being made is that a sound structure alone cannot achieve desired outcomes but that process deserves particular attention.

This study has sought to examine the effectiveness of process in joint working arrangements between local authorities and groups such as the voluntary sector, and their effects. In general we found that closer working with the authority was welcomed by the voluntary and private sectors, and more particularly that the setting up of forums was seen as a positive step in this direction. Likewise, involvement in political processes such as an Under Eights sub-committee was seen as an acknowledgement of the contribution of other players by an authority. This being so, there were however negative comments, mainly around issues of participation and empowerment. These have already been raised in relation to the section 19 Reviews above, but are illustrated most clearly in the case of Authority A, where the issue was looked at in greater detail in the case studies (cf. Bull et al., 1994b).

In this authority, careful consideration had been given to drawing the voluntary and private sectors into the process of early years policy development. There were representatives from these sectors on the Early Years Sub-Committee (with a voice but no voting rights), and the forum system sought to secure wide representation from them, community interests and parents. Officers responsible were committed to the principles of co-ordination and joint working, and felt they had made great strides in that direction. They seemed unaware that representatives of the voluntary and private sectors on those structures were less than satisfied with the process, and why. But this became clear in the course of the case study.

The first example of ineffective process concerns the working of the Sub-Committee. In interview, a co-opted member from the voluntary sector spoke of a situation that was dominated by procedures and regulations which were not explained to her, and which was very formal. She went on:

*I never felt welcome there, it's so cliquey...I have never really been introduced... I feel like I don't know if I had the courage to speak up and ask something... didn't feel it very good at all, ...very intimidating. I felt it might make me look silly, make us feel silly. Even people [officers] I know very well ... – they all ignored me.*

Similar problems were encountered in the county early years forum. The same representative commented that 'sometimes when professionals get together it's very difficult ... volunteers sometimes don't understand'. Her feelings were echoed by another representative on these bodies:'X goes [to the meetings]...She feels intimidated. ..[they are] talking above her head most of the time'.

A second issue relates to the content and success of forum meetings. Commenting on an early meeting, a private sector representative observed it was 'most boring, they spent the meeting redrafting a document prepared at the last meeting'. Similar comments were made by two voluntary sector representatives:

*XX:At one point 'Y' said that going to the meetings was a waste of time–*

*XY:I think we've all felt like that...*

Issues relating to process were raised in other authorities too, and mainly concern representation on and the role of forums:

*[They]...can be quite elitist...We would like to see more ethnic minority people ..more people on low incomes coming along (northern county)*

*Many networks exist...[but they] could be more formally set up (metropolitan borough)*

*[We]...ought to be able to make a much more positive contribution than commenting on a presentation made by the local authority (London borough)*

Three main issues concerning process are highlighted above. The first relates to the designated role of forums. Where a local authority constitutes and defines the role of a forum, it is possible that this might be at variance with the wishes of its membership, as illustrated in the London borough quoted above. Secondly, and again within a model where a local authority takes the lead in setting up and running a forum, the membership may perceive it to be lacking in terms of representativeness, or structure, or other aspect. Such a situation should not arise in the NEYN model, where the forum's terms of reference and its constitution are defined by its members. It could also be avoided in the other model if the local authority does not dictate the forum's terms of reference, if all members are accorded equal status in deciding on the terms of reference, and the process allows this.

A third issue concerns content and ownership of meetings of the various co-ordinating and consultative bodies. It was seen in Authority A that the procedures, language and conduct of its sub-committee meetings had an intimidating effect on outsiders such as co-opted members. It seems evident that if participation on these bodies is to be more than just nominal, special efforts need to be made to explain procedures and otherwise put members at ease. But while sub-committee meetings can be expected to follow established procedures, the work of the forum in the model followed by Authority A should have been open to question by its members. Yet comments quoted above make it plain that they felt themselves to be participating in a meeting generated by the local authority rather than themselves: while they were unhappy with the proceedings, they did not intervene to change it.

The concerns raised above lie at the heart of issues around participation and empowerment, where empowerment involves giving people a voice for articulating their needs. In the final analysis, the question would be whether the co-ordinating / consultative mechanisms function to serve the purposes of the authority, or whether they represent a movement towards genuine involvement of outside interests in the process of policy formulation. If it is the latter, local authorities will need to be aware that this involves more than inviting their participation on coordinating bodies. Taking the argument to its extreme, inviting formal participation of non-statutory sector representatives on co-ordinating bodies, but then leaving the process of participation opaque, can be experienced as tokenistic and, at worst, disempowering.

*External constraints*

While the Children Act and Guidance advocate closer working relations between agencies in developing early childhood services, external factors and influences have militated against co-ordinated working. In particular, the NHS and Community Care Act 1990 saw the breakup of health authorities into health trusts and along purchaser / provider lines, disrupting established working links and making identification of individuals with whom to form new links difficult for some time. Similarly, impending local government reorganisation meant that long-term planning for service development was made difficult for some county councils. Likewise the 1988 Education Reform Act which introduced local management of schools led to reorganisations with severe reductions in staffing for many education authorities; and again, difficulties in identifying staff to undertake the Review duty with social services officers. Co-ordination, with the implication of some loss of autonomy, was not easy in this climate, as succinctly described by an officer from a county authority:

> *Education departments everywhere feel very threatened by central government cuts.. It leads to defensiveness and protecting territory. I think at the highest officer level in this county there is unwillingness to let anyone else in.*

Additionally, the financial climate was also changing. While some authorities received a favourable budget settlement, others experienced severe budget cuts. An extreme example of how budgetary constraints could lead to a complete breakdown in co-ordination is provided by Authority B.

At the first stage of our study it was found that Authority B demonstrated a commitment to co-ordinated working. A high provider of services, the model of co-ordination it had developed covered local authority departments only, and did not extend to outside interests such as the independent sector and other statutory bodies. Early years co-ordinating structures were at a policy development level, and consisted of a Members Group comprising members from the main provider Committees; an Early Years Strategy Group comprising senior and chief officers from the main providing departments and the central executive; and a Children Act Review Group comprising senior officers only, from the same departments.

Once policy had been agreed within these groups, implementation was the responsibility of individual departments; with senior officers providing a focal point for the two-way flow of information. Routine grass-roots level feedback was gained mainly through a system of support/discussion groups for each of the provider-types in the borough, organised and facilitated by officers from the different departments.

The authority agreed its early years strategy, and completed its first section 19 Review on schedule, in which was included a directory of services for children aged under eight and an action plan with specific targets. But the process of arriving at these was hampered at every stage by departmental rivalries, exacerbated by a worsening financial situation. Financial constraints had resulted in a series of major re-structurings, with substantial job losses, and a merging of some departments. A rationalisation of service delivery was being considered. A proposal to move all day care services for children aged under eight to the education authority was bitterly resented by the other providing departments, and seen by senior officers as reflecting the power relations between chief officers rather than any other considerations. These perceptions permeated the working of both the Strategy Group and the Review Group.

By the final fieldwork stage, co-ordination had broken down completely. While the Strategy Group had completed its task, the Review Group which should have been overseeing the implementation of the action plan and carrying forward the next Review, had disbanded, due to acrimonious relations between officers. Responsibility for most of the authority's services for young children had been moved to education; and there were no formal working links between education and social services. The action plan of the first Review had been implemented, but mainly through the efforts of the officer from the policy unit, who has since left the service of the authority. No-one had been identified to lead the second Review.

**Evaluation of the Act**

In evaluating a local authority's co-ordination function under the Children Act, it is important to remember that co-ordinating services is, by definition, no easy task. Apart from the external constraints outlined above, it involves some loss of autonomy for the organisations concerned, and a need for negotiation, compromise, trust and mutual respect in order to achieve desired objectives. Additionally, while the rhetoric is not new, co-ordination in practice is relatively new in the field of services for young children.

The purpose of co-ordination suggested in the Act and Guidance is to produce more efficient, comprehensive and holistic services and to avoid fragmentation and overlap. In other words, the hope is that through joint working, agencies can achieve more than 'the sum of their separate parts'. This chapter has focused on the structures and processes used by local authorities towards this end.

Firstly, there has been recent growth in co-ordinating structures which represents an adherence to the principle of co-ordination at policy level.

While this may have been at least in part a result of mandated co-ordination in response to the Act, comments such as 'chief officers now speak with one voice', and 'there's a willingness to co-ordinate on the part of key players inside and outside the local authority', which were not isolated examples, suggests that the benefits of co-ordinated working have been acknowledged in many authorities. All authorities with interdepartmental co-ordinating structures perceived the process of joint working to be in itself beneficial: it had built dialogue where little existed before. As highlighted in the literature and demonstrated in the case studies, bridging professional divides can be painful, but engaging in dialogue is an essential first step that could lead to an appreciation of the complementary roles each plays in a child's development, and thus to a more holistic approach to service provision. At the same time, the experience of Authority C indicates that professional allegiances can be persistent and disruptive of co-ordination processes; and points to a need for dialogue to be continuing and to extend to all levels of management.

Secondly, most authorities had acted on Guidance advice to develop links with the private and voluntary sectors among others. Opening up the policy development process to include such interests can be seen as an acknowledgement by the local authority that they could contribute positively to it, and a move away from the previous top-down approach to service planning. Comments from representatives of these interests from many different authorities confirm that they feel themselves to be more valued by their respective authorities by such an inclusion. Here again communication has been enhanced, and this together with the better working relations it has engendered must be seen as a positive outcome of co-ordination. At the same time authorities need to guard against the danger of considering only *organised* interests in the field.

Inclusion of voluntary and private sector interests in the decision-making process was seen to be at two levels: (i) the political, and more usually, (ii) through use of forums. At the political level, co-opting unelected members onto committees or sub-committees can be interpreted as part of a wider political process, not specific to early years/children's services or the Children Act, but more to political outlook and style of local government. The work of committees is seen to be the responsibility of elected members alone in some authorities, and not inconsistent with a policy of working in co-ordination with the independent sector. Indeed, it is possible to envisage a system whereby policy recommendations are made to a committee by a lower-level body such as a forum, in which those interests are represented. Provided sufficient attention is given to effective process, and provided such recommendations are given due consideration, such a system could form a model of good practice, and work to mutual benefit.

Thirdly, the section 19 review is the instrument designed by the Act and Guidance for achieving more co-ordinated services. The statutory duty to review services imposed on social services departments and local education authorities has compelled the two departments to work together, though not to the same extent in the different authorities. In some cases it was the impetus for co-ordinated working. The first stage of our study indicated that the first reviews had mainly been a mapping exercise, and through which gaps in provision had been identified, but the project was completed too early for the achievements of the second reviews to be included in this evaluation. However, the reviews were almost universally recognised as having raised the profile of services for young children. But if the intention is to provide quality services which are responsive to the needs of the community, the consultation process requires to be carefully thought out and implemented. Whilst forums provide a good mechanism for this purpose, they should not be the only form of consultation, because, as pointed out earlier, they often represent organised interests only. Other forms of consultation need to be developed to ensure that less influential voices, such as minority ethnic interests can also be heard. But in the final analysis, without political backing for the review and its recommendations the end result cannot easily be achieved.

Finally, the concept of co-ordination as outlined in the Children Act and Guidance can itself be evaluated. The Act and Guidance recommend that local authorities work 'in partnership' with voluntary and private sector and community interests in developing services, but the power imbalance in the relationship has not been addressed. For, a local authority and its officers carry the status and authority of government, which puts them on a different footing from voluntary and private sector providers and community interests. While this does not imply that the latter are powerless it does make for an unequal partnership in many cases. Similarly, whilst recognising the limitations of a system of service provision developed in parallel by different departments, and therefore recommending a co-ordinated approach to service provision, the Act and Guidance continue to perpetuate the divisions represented by them by referring to social services and education departments as 'the two authorities' rather than two departments of a local authority. However, the Act did represent some attempt to promote cohesion by recommending a corporate approach to the development of early years policy, but the implications of this recommendation were not addressed in the Act or Guidance. For while education and social services are split off conceptually and operationally at national level, both with their own agendas, it will be difficult for cohesion at the local level to rise much above the level of rhetoric. In the absence of a national policy on services for young children, this situation is likely to remain unchanged. These issues are discussed more fully in the concluding chapter of this book.

**Lessons from the Research**

- Overcoming professional boundaries is a first step in successful co-ordination or integration of services. Professionals need to move beyond the traditional care–education–play divide to an appreciation of the complementary roles each other play in a child's development, and through which a 'common language' can be found.

- Different models of co-ordination can be chosen by different authorities, reflecting factors such as political outlook and style of government in the authority. There is a need for the chosen model to be compatible with the authority's style of government.

- If the model chosen includes the involvement of independent sector representatives and other interested parties, the authority needs to ensure that co-ordinating structures allow for less influential voices to be heard. It may prove necessary to foster the participation of more marginal groups on local forums to achieve that objective.

- Opening up the process of policy formulation to local interest groups and provider organisations involves more than inviting their participation on co-ordinating bodies. Local authorities need to be aware that factors such as its procedures and the language and conduct of its meetings could be unfamiliar and intimidating to outsiders. Unless they take steps to overcome these problems, the participation of such groups could remain marginal.

- Special measures will need to be taken to consult with minority ethnic groups in the development of services. Local authorities may find the checklist developed by SIA (Qaiyoom, 1992) a useful tool in consulting with such community groups.

CHAPTER

# 4 The Registration and Inspection of Day Care Services

**Julie Bull**

## Background

The regulation of services for young children has a long history. The Nurseries and Child-minders Regulation Act of 1948 preceded the Children Act 1989 and though there is not much systematic information about how previous legislation worked in practice, the need for reform had been long called for (Elfer and Beasely, 1991). The Act introduced a new 'modernised registration system' which now provides the framework for the provision of day care services for children aged under eight. This part of the legislation extends beyond local authorities' welfare role towards children 'in need' and so potentially impacts on the majority of children under eight who attend some form of day care service. As such, the new regulatory regime was one of the more far-reaching and controversial policy changes in relation to day care services included in the Children Act.

The key aspects of the new system were:

- criteria on who is a 'fit person' to provide day care;
- a framework of mandatory requirements regarding staff: child ratios, health and safety of premises and equipment, and record keeping;
- the statutory requirement to re-register all existing provision under the new framework within the first year of the Act's implementation;
- the introduction of annual inspection for day care services registered under the Act;
- the inclusion of out-of-school and holiday provision for school aged children under eight within the new regulatory regime;
- an emphasis on the need for providers to pay attention to matters of cultural, ethnic and linguistic diversity, and for local authorities to regulate this as part of the inspection process.

The objectives of the duty placed on local authorities to regulate standards in day care are outlined in Guidance, and include ensuring services meet acceptable standards and are provided within an agreed framework (DoH 1991, para. 4.9). Elsewhere in Guidance, the objective of providing a mechanism for ensuring quality of care is repeatedly implied. Paragraphs 6.24–6.38, for example, offer a wide-ranging discussion of factors influencing 'quality of care' of which inspectors should be mindful and it is also suggested that the registration process should function to 'help the setting up of good quality services' (ibid.: para 4.9). To this extent, the objectives of the new regime are ambiguously articulated and it remains unclear whether minimum standards or quality (however defined) are the desired outcome of the new regulations. One of the principles underlying good practice in day care, as outlined in Guidance, is that 'children's welfare and development are paramount' (ibid.: para 6.2) but this does not constitute the legal principle of paramountcy which underpins the parts of the Act which relate to the decisions of social workers or courts; it is only general advice.

Circular LAC (93)1, issued subsequently, goes on to suggest the regulatory role must be approached flexibly by local authorities in the light of local needs for the expansion of services. It states that local authorities should not be setting standards that are 'unrealistically high to the point where they inhibit expansion'. The Circular removed the need for extensive police checks on those working in services, and amended the original statement about the need for qualifications among staff. While clearly welcomed by some service providers, other provider organisations and commentators have seen the circular as a weakening of the system as originally envisaged (Elfer, 1993).

The case brought against the London Borough of Sutton in their attempt to enforce a no smacking policy in registration of childminders in line with advice in Guidance, which clearly advises against physical forms of punishment, has further reinforced the point that Guidance is not legally prescriptive. It also introduces another element into the quality/expansion dilemma: local authorities must balance their requirements with the needs and wishes of parents. The Government has taken the view that where parents make a private arrangement with a childminder or other day care provider about discipline, which includes permitting smacking as a means of last resort, then that is a matter for the parents. In this context, Circular LAC (94)23 qualifies the advice in Guidance, making it clear that this advice is not prescriptive, should not be applied too rigidly and must be read as a whole.

In managing their regulatory role therefore, local authorities are asked to balance a number of potentially competing policy objectives: the protection of the welfare of children; the continued supply of services which are accessible to parents; the provision of services at an appropriate standard; and the respect for parental wishes and responsibilities. No relative priority is given to any of these objectives; it is suggested that local authorities can meet them all through achieving the 'right balance'. Further, the intended outcome, in terms of what standards are to be expected of providers, remains fluid, particularly in the light of the need for flexibility, stressed in Circular LAC (93)1.

**The Wider Debate**

The strengthened role of local authorities as regulators, rather than providers, of services in the early years reflects broader trends in social policy. The provision of 'personal social services' has proliferated in the private and informal sector, and has been accompanied by greater public powers of regulation at a central level. The NHS and Community Care Act 1990 was pivotal in reinforcing the role of local authorities as purchasers and regulators of services in a 'mixed economy' of care. The Children Act, while retaining a role in provision for local authorities, both echoed these trends and, in terms of implementation, has been influenced by developments in the organisation and delivery of social services brought about by community care reforms.

In particular, the establishment of independent inspection units which followed the community care reforms, provided an organisational model for the inspection of children's services, which many local authorities have adopted with the introduction of the Children Act. To date, there has been no clear statement from the Department of Health as to whether this is considered the most appropriate structure for children's services. The regulation and inspection of social services as a whole, including day care services for children aged under eight, are also now the subject of a Review consultation exercise, which considers, among other issues, alternative models for regulating services, including self regulation, and the establishment of a national inspectorate (DoH, 1995b). Among practitioners there remains a debate about the location of regulation in relation to the support and development of services for young children and about the degree of specialism required of those inspecting services for young children.

It may be seen as paradoxical that in pursuing a commitment to reduce state intervention in the public provision of personal social services, it has been necessary to strengthen powers to regulate them. In fact, public funding for day care services has always been low and the bulk of provision has been located in the independent sector in the form of childminders, private day nurseries and playgroups (see chapter 1). Currently, there is a critique of regulation which originates in the sphere of industry but has now been extended to the social care field, which has led 'the Government [to have] a fundamental commitment to reduce the burden of regulation on businesses, charities and individuals' (Hunter Johnston, 1996: 2). While quality assurance regimes form a dominant theme in the new ethos of public sector management and have been the concern of social services departments in their new enabling role, a parallel political debate has been concerned with the inhibiting effects of regulations on the private market. The reaction to the new regulations and the concern about the effects of regulation on the growing sector of private business involved in the provision of day care, as expressed in Circular LAC (93)1, reflect the strong influence of this debate.

The most recent policy initiative in services for young children is the current proposal to introduce a voucher scheme for the parents of all four year olds which will be redeemable in a variety of settings. Accompanying this initiative will be a review of the current inspection regimes, in an attempt to harmonise the framework currently operational under the Children Act and OFSTED inspection of schools. There will be a new emphasis, brought about by the new 'light touch' inspection regime which emerges from this, on the desirable outcomes for learning among this age group of children and a consultation document has outlined various proposals for incorporating a new inspection framework into those already in operation.

The professional debate about the nature of quality in services for young children has a longer history and extends beyond the issue of regulation. Balaguer et al. (1991), for example, suggest that regulation is only one element of creating the conditions needed to ensure quality which is ultimately a relative and value-based concept. The pay, training and conditions of workers in the services comprise essential elements of quality of care which are only touched upon, if addressed at all, in the duty to regulate services introduced in the Children Act.

In short, there are a number of different strands which form the context to current policy on regulating day care services. Key issues centre on how much regulation is appropriate and what form it should take: is the role of regulation to set minimum standards, to promote quality or protect children? Underlying such questions are other issues: whose interests does the regulator serve and what weight should be given to the different stake-holders involved? Who are the 'consumers' of early childhood services, children or their parents? Can day care services be treated as businesses and what does this imply for the welfare of the children who attend them? These strands involve a wide range of interest groups, including politicians, policy-makers, professionals, proprietors of private day care services, parents and children. Whether the proliferation of concerns within this wider debate add up to any form of consensus is doubtful, but provides an important context in which to evaluate whether this part of the Children Act can be said to have achieved the original objectives it contained.

## Implementation Three Years after the Act

*Organisational structures*

The largest group of authorities in the sample (8/17) had incorporated the inspection of children's services into *inspection units* working on a model of 'arms length' inspection to a greater or lesser degree. Six of the authorities studied had *day care* or *under eights teams* within the mainstream social services departments or within newly established 'integrated service' departments. A further three authorities operated some kind of 'dual system'; in two cases they had both an inspection unit and a day care team which inspected different types of day care services, in one registration and inspection was split between a team in social services and an inspection unit. This represented little movement over the two years since the stage one visits, other than two authorities launching new 'integrated under eights services'.

The two main groups of organisational structure found both between and sometimes within authorities (inspection units and day care teams) represented different practical and conceptual 'models' of the regulatory task in relation to day care services. Where day care services had been brought within inspection units as part of the implementation of the Children Act, it was usually rationalised in terms of streamlining, standardising and, most importantly, separating out inspection from the provision, support and development of services. Where existing arrangements of regulation provided within locally based teams were continued, the combination of the support and development function underpinned the organisational style. Box 4.1 shows how the contrast in the values and in the view of day care services which was reflected within the two main organisational models in their pure form could be characterised.

**Box 4.1**

**Values and view of day care services in two main organisational models for regulation of day care services**

| Inspection units | Day care or other SSD teams |
|---|---|
| Objective approach | Based on relationship with providers |
| Arms length | Local |
| Support role separate | Support as integral |
| 'Policing' role | Supportive role |
| One-off | On-going |
| Day care as private market; LA as regulator only | Day care as a public/community resource; LA as enabler/provider |

In practice however, the local authorities studied here rarely conformed to the pure models suggested by such a dichotomous characterisation. For example, only one authority conformed to the pure model of an inspection unit with a clearly delineated boundary between inspection and support. Otherwise, within the inspection units, there was considerable diversity with three adopting a formal support role to include such tasks as running duty advice systems to providers, offering training to providers, and making visits additional to annual inspections. Other authorities without a formal support role also reported some involvement with support work, even if this was limited. In implementing the new regulation system, therefore, most authorities appear to have found the boundary between regulation and support difficult to draw, and have become involved in support work to varying degrees. The level of support work undertaken in different authorities differentiates them beyond a simple contrast between arm's length or other organisational models.

But although the distinction between the two organisational styles is not as sharp as suggested in the model, differences in emphasis based on the dimensions it charts were reflected in the local authorities in the study.

At the extreme ends of a continuum, different regulatory cultures could be identified; one conforming to a more top-down form of inspection than the other, more developmental approach.

The views sought from regulation managers and staff on whether regulation should include or be separate from a support/development role also revealed polarised positions. Those in favour of combining support and development gave the following reasons for their view:

- The need for support work to raise standards.
- The need to 'follow through' on issues raised in inspection.
- The need to develop good practice.
- The need to build up a relationship with providers and to work with them, especially in childminding.
- The need for a knowledge base and overview of local services.
- Less confusion for providers than two different functions.
- Support is the more interesting part of the job.
- Support has to come from somewhere and there's no-one else to do it.

Those in favour of separating the two functions gave the following in support of their position:

- More consistency and objectivity can be achieved.
- There is no potential for conflict of interest.
- You are not inspecting your own work.
- Roles and expectations are clearer on both sides, and so there is less confusion for service providers.
- Enforcement of standards is easier, including the option of litigation.

Most staff were largely in support of the organisational style and culture in which they currently worked, although some staff in inspection units wanted to do more support work, and some staff working in day care teams experienced some conflict in their combined role. Most were in favour of combining some element of support with their regulatory role, but the term 'support' encompassed a variety of meanings from simply acting as a point of contact for service providers, to offering training, ongoing advice and making drop-in visits. In practice, the amount of support work undertaken by registration officers was determined as much by the amount of time they had available as by how they conceptualised the relationship between regulation and support (see chapter 5). This was true in both inspection units and day care teams.

*Resources*

It was extremely difficult to compare the resources available for regulation between different authorities, partly because of differences in the way the task was defined in terms of support and also because in three authorities, inspection staff were 'generic', i.e. they also inspected services for adults. Additional complicating factors were the unknown quantity of out-of-school services in most authorities and different levels of managerial and administrative support. With these caveats in mind, a crude measure of workload – a workload index[3] – was applied to each local author-

**Figure 4.1: Regulation staffing and workload in the sample authorities**

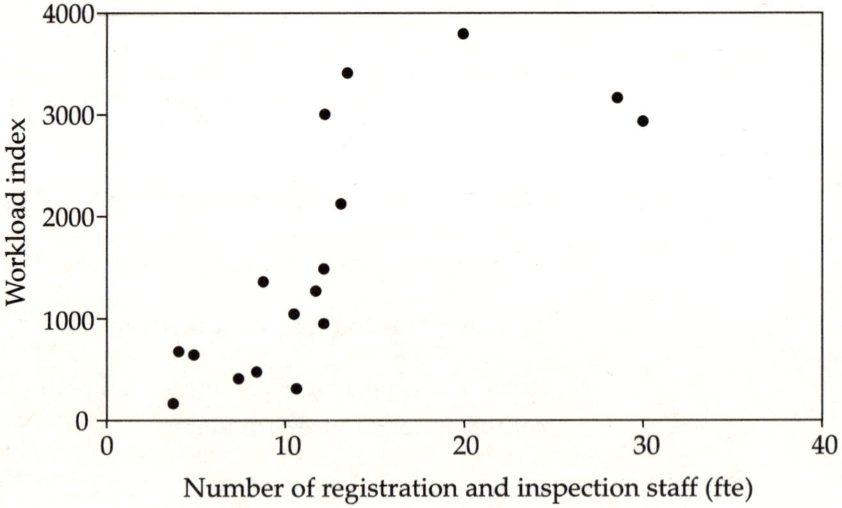


3. The workload index is based on counting day nurseries as 3 workload units, playgroups as 2 units and childminders as 1 unit, and applying these weightings to the number of registered services in each local authority. The weightings are based on data from the service providers' survey, which recorded average lengths of inspections for different provider types.

ity to provide some indication of the extent of disparities in staffing resources. This exercise, the results of which are shown in figure 4.1, reveals very different levels of staffing between local authorities.

The other 'measure' of the resourcing of the regulatory function is the perceptions of staff themselves, as reported in the third stage interviews. This data revealed that while most regulation managers (12/19) described staffing levels as adequate, many of them qualified this by saying they were only adequate to perform their statutory duties. Over half the regulation officers (29/54) interviewed perceived staffing levels to be 'inadequate'. There appeared to be some relationship between organisational structure and perceptions of staffing levels; staff in day care teams in social services departments (not in integrated services) were less likely to report inadequate staffing levels than those in inspection units or integrated services. Eleven of the 17 authorities had a workload formula as recommended in Guidance. Workload formulae were more common in inspection units than in local teams or integrated services.

Although perceptions of workload varied within, as well as between, authorities, there were seven authorities where most staff reported inadequate staffing levels, indicating chronic and persistent problems of workload. Some of these problems were in part explained by factors specific to the authority, such as a strike which occurred at the time of implementation, reorganisation, and evident managerial failure. However, some of these were attributable only to apparently low levels of staffing – the authorities who appeared in this category were, for the most part, also those who appeared at the lower end of the staffing workload index. Some of the authorities with apparently severe problems of workload also had a workload formula, although it may have been based on inaccurate estimates of levels of provision, or not even operationalised. This raises some questions about the adequacy and effectiveness of workload formulae.

The consequences of inadequate staffing levels, particularly in the groups of authorities identified above, were manifold. Most obviously, six authorities mentioned workload backlogs – in one of these no annual inspections had yet begun, in another officers were aiming to complete only 30 per cent of annual inspections that year, in another inspections were continuing alongside outstanding re-registration of services. The most frequently cited of the other consequences were: the loss of the support function; poor staff morale and stress among staff; the limitations on the rigour with which inspections could be carried out; inspection reports to providers being delayed, and the inability to pick up and follow through on concerns about particular providers; and damaged relationships with service providers.

Although some local authorities had severe workload difficulties and a great many others clearly felt overstretched, most registration officers (35/54) were managing to complete at least one annual inspection of all services and complete new registrations within the timescales recommended in the Guidance (6 months for full day care and 3 months for other day care providers).

*Standards and process*

Most authorities in the sample had changed the guidelines on standards for providers over the first three years of implementation or were in the process of doing so. Where the changes were substantive, this was most usually in response to either Circular LAC (93)1, or the Sutton judgement, or both. More widely reported however, was a shift in emphasis or style brought about by these developments, rather than a tangible change in policy as formally stated. The most significant outcome of the shifts brought about by Circular LAC (93)1 was a sense of caution among authorities about enforcing standards to the point of litigation. This caution operated at several levels of the inspection process: in the ways in which officers 'self-censored' their own decisions, and in the amount of backing they received at a managerial, legal and political level for taking action against providers who were not complying with standards. While nearly all authorities defined themselves as flexible in their approach to regulation, Circular LAC (93)1 had called into question the limits of flexibility, the parameters of decision making, the minimum standard beyond which standards could not drop. In this sense, Circular LAC (93)1 was seen to have undermined what was originally perceived as a clear framework of standards, with some damage to credibility with providers. Officers reported nursery owners exploiting the exhortation to be flexible as a way of not complying with basic standards on numbers of children in a facility.

A related consequence of this was on staff morale. One officer summed up the response to the Circular thus:

> *the difference is in how we feel about our work. We thought we had more power or control but the Circular took this away. Now we don't feel able to do anything about less adequate services.*

The response to the Sutton judgement had been either to maintain a no-smacking policy which had been in operation before the judgement and to wait for it to be challenged, or to review existing practice and to require parental consent from childminders who intended to smack. Most officers however, stressed the support of service providers themselves, most pertinently in this case, childminders, for no-smacking policies. Although many authorities continued to advise against the practice of physical forms of discipline, the status of this advice was felt to be such that potential service providers could not be refused registration on this ground alone.

Not all officers however, thought that the impact of the Circular and Sutton case had been negative. A minority thought that the call for flexibility contained in Circular LAC (93)1 was appropriate and necessary, particularly for under-resourced playgroups, and interpreted the Circular to be an endorsement of an approach which was supportive and developmental.

An important feature of the new regulation system introduced by the Act was the statutory duty to inspect services once they are registered. It is for local authorities to decide if additional visits are made to service providers or the number of visits required for one inspection. Over half of the authorities (10/17) in the sample made no extra visits, except where there were problems, although sometimes there appeared to be variation in this practice among individual officers. A small group of authorities (3/17) made additional visits to providers in certain categories, such as new groups, or providers where concerns had been raised at annual inspection. Some authorities made several visits during the process of registration of new providers, or two visits as part of the inspection process. In another small group of authorities (4/17), more than one visit to providers was routinely carried out as a matter of policy. For example, in one authority staff visited childminders three times a year, while in another authority staff made three-monthly 'review visits' and one visit per month to childminders used by social services for children 'in need'. In yet another authority although regular additional visits were the intention of policy they rarely happened in practice because of the pressure to meet statutory inspection demands.

Additional visits were made for both 'policing' or monitoring purposes and more commonly, in the interests of supporting service providers. Whether they were undertaken or not depended on the structure of the regulation function in an authority, i.e whether or not it sought to combine regulation with support. Additional visits were more likely if these functions were combined. It also depended to large degree on workload and resources and was therefore unlikely to occur in those authorities where the levels of staffing were relatively low. Nearly all regulation officers, regardless of the organisational model in which they worked, would like to have made more than one visit to providers and gave the pressure of workload as the reason they could not. Serious concerns were raised by some about the adequacy of one visit in ensuring standards were met; as one officer put it 'providers can put their house in order for one announced visit, but we don't know what could be happening in between'.

- The duration of inspection visits themselves differed according to type of service. In the service providers survey, for example, data revealed that inspection of day nurseries took longer on average than either those of playgroups or childminders, and childminder inspections were on average shorter than both other provider types (Moss et al., 1995; table 4). An analysis of inspection reports and documentation, collected in the final visits to authorities also indicates that inspection of childminders is a less complex process and was less likely to involve detailed observation of interaction between the minder and children – despite the fact that childminders are the most isolated and least publicly visible day care providers.

Inspection documents also varied in their format, style and content. Some authorities adopted more of a 'checklist approach' while others allowed for more open-ended discussion and judgement by the inspecting officer. Some inspection reports took the form of a handwritten completed pro forma, some were reports compiled after the actual inspection which used common headings. The attention given to good practice issues and those relating to 'quality of care' was evidently greater in some authorities than others, while the treatment of more tangible issues of space standards and health and safety issues was more constant. One example of variation in practices concerned the way in which equal opportunities issues were handled within inspection documentation. This could involve the use of one 'catch all' question on inspection forms or pre-inspection questionnaires such as the following example from an outer London borough's inspection format:

> *In what ways do you ensure that children in your care have equal opportunities? (A space of one line is allowed for the reply)*

This could be compared with authorities whose formats contained a series of questions relating to issues of diversity, under a separate heading, or in one case, an authority which dealt with both gender and cultural diversity separately and in some detail. For the most part, questions of diversity seemed to focus on 'race', rather than on gender or other equal opportunity issues.

Questions about care practice generally took a question and answer format. Relatively few examples were found of types of questions which seemed designed to encourage a reflexive response from practitioners, rather than one in which there was an implicitly 'correct' answer. The following example from an inner London authority is one such exception:

> *Think of a situation where a child had responded a) well to your handling and b) not so well.*

Grasping the nuances of difference in regulatory styles however, is an elusive task. Documentation alone does not reflect the actual processes involved with great accuracy which may involve lengthy but unrecorded discussion with providers. For the process to be more fully understood, a more systematic observation of the inspection process in different authorities would be required.

Perhaps the greatest area of professional judgement required of regulation officers is in the assessment of whether someone is a 'fit person' to provide day care, which is central in the registration process. Guidance offers criteria on which local authorities are to base such judgements which include tangible issues such as health, experience with children, known involvement in criminal cases involving children and so on. However, these criteria also include the prospective provider's ability to provide 'warm and consistent care', their knowledge of and attitude to multi-cultural issues and people of different racial origins, and their commitment to treat all children as individuals and with equal concern. Clearly, these involve officers in judgements of a much more qualitative kind. Local authorities had developed some identifiable, though different, strategies for approaching the issue of fitness:

- The first could be characterised as relying largely on 'the checklist approach' in which the core of the assessment was that of police, health checks and personal references.

- The second approach was that which relied principally on discussion with the prospective provider as a way of probing and attempting to change attitudes, on issues of diversity for example.

- The third approach attempted to standardise the criteria on which the assessment was made in a 'fit person interview' with discussion taking place under set headings. One authority conducted such an interview on council premises.

Although seven authorities had developed 'fit person' interview criteria, most relied on a mixture of the first and second approach summed up by one officer as 'a combination of checklist, gut feeling and experience'. Sometimes differences in approach were discernible within as well as between authorities on this issue. One of the difficulties highlighted by officers about the assessment was that they made it before observation with children was possible. This made the assessment of a person's ability to provide warm and consistent care particularly difficult. Also frequently mentioned was a concern that providers knew the right answers to give at the point of registration but that this did not reflect their practice in reality and this again raised the need for the monitoring of standards of care to be more on-going than was usually possible.

In general, there was a range of attitudes to the assessment of fitness. Some adopted a legalistic attitude which identified fitness as the absence of evidence to the contrary, as expressed by these officers:

*We're not assessing fitness, we're having to prove if they're unfit.*

*We're not really checking whether they're a fit person, we're more ticking off the points that they're not.*

*We assume they're fit unless we have proof otherwise.*

Others perceived the assessment as a highly discretionary aspect of their job, relying more on subjective assessments than procedures, but presenting them with little to stand on as a basis for refusing or cancelling registration as summed up by the following quotes;

*A lot is subjective or 'gut instinct'. It's very difficult to prove people are or not adequate so we have to register people who are bordering on unsuitable.*

*The fit person criteria are very sketchy, very open. This allows for professional judgement by day care advisers and you learn a lot through discussion especially at the first visit, but you can't assess warm and consistent care until you see them in practice by which time they're already registered. You can't refuse registration on the basis of a feeling...it's the same with equal opportunities – they say the right things but you get a feeling.*

What is clear is that, inherent in the registration and inspection process, there is considerable scope for professional discretion or judgement on the part of regulation officers and that this demands a range of skills and experience from them, including awareness of multi-cultural issues, negotiating and interviewing and inspection skills and report writing, as well as some knowledge of the kind of issues involved in early years education and care. In reality, staff undertaking this task came from a variety of backgrounds and were variously qualified. The most common qualification held by registration officers was the NNEB; half of those interviewed were qualified in this way. Nine had some kind of social work background (CQSW or CSS) and three held a teaching qualification. Other qualifications mentioned and often held in addition to those already given were the PPA diploma and BTEC certificate. Only four officers had no qualifications relating to children. Nearly every officer interviewed had experience of working in services for young children.

The grades and pay of registration officers, reflecting their professional status, varied considerably between local authorities. While some of these staff were offered a wide range of in-service training, others had far fewer training opportunities. For example, one authority, a large county with an inspection unit, had a planned annual programme of training for registration officers based on their perceived training needs. In the twelve months prior to being interviewed officers had attended courses on a variety of topics related to their work including inspection skills, report writing, counselling and dealing with complaints. By contrast, in another authority, also a large county with an inspection unit, none of the four registration officers interviewed (all from an NNEB background) had training in inspection skills, and they had attended only one in-service training course (on complaints) in the previous 12 months. One officer described the situation of registration officers as one with 'no career structure, no management and no training'. Staff in this authority had been redeployed to an inspection unit as part of Children Act implementation and clearly felt unsupported in making the transition to what they perceived to be a new working ethos.

In only six authorities had some training in inspection skills been provided for registration officers. Not surprisingly therefore, inspection skills and also equal opportunities were the most frequently identified training needs among registration officers. Child protection and using the law / dealing with complaints were the next most frequently cited training needs of officers. This need for training, especially in inspection skills and equal opportunities, has also been found by the National Children's Bureau who have reported that 'frontline officers particularly need training in how to implement the requirements of the Children Act to pay attention to equal opportunities issues...and referred to the need for negotiating skills and the ability to tease out a standard in the registration and inspection process' (McQuail and Pugh, 1995: 103).

Given the apparent differences between authorities on many aspects of their approach to registration and inspection (also noted by McQuail and Pugh (1995) in their study), the question of consistency is clearly raised. Many authorities felt however, that the Children Act, both in terms of standards and in terms of organisation, had gone a long way to improving the consistency of the process. In larger counties in particular, consistency of approach within authorities remained a major issue and was monitored though supervision, team meetings, 'case-swapping', and regular audits of samples of inspection reports.

*Using the law*

There were few recorded cases of refusal or cancellation of registration. Eight of the 17 authorities, for example had no such cases to report, although one had a current case of cancellation pending. Only three authorities had more than five cases to report. Of the eight authorities who had taken no cases to the point of cancelling or refusing registration, two were inspection units. In the small group of three authorities who had more than five recorded cases, two were inspection units and one had a dual team/inspection unit structure split according to service type. On the basis of this there is some evidence to suggest that local authorities with inspection units seemed more likely to have taken cases than those with teams who also provided support to providers, but the association is not strong. The association which does exist may be explained as an inhibiting effect of the conflict of interest involved in combining the two roles. Alternatively, it could be viewed as a positive consequence of adopting a supportive rather than legalistic regulatory style.

All of the cases of cancellation or refusal of registration had involved either childminders or day nurseries, rather than playgroups. Some of the cases had been brought reactively, i.e. in response to complaints or allegations from a third party, while some action had arisen as part of the inspection process. The most common ground under which providers had been refused registration was on 'fitness', either of the prospective provider or of a person on the premises, particularly regarding child protection issues. Most of these cases involved a record of concern about child abuse in the past or some evidence of risk of child abuse in the future. Only one case, concerning full-time day care, involved what could be termed 'good practice issues' where poor interaction between staff and children was given as part of the case against the service provider together with concerns about previous convictions and complaints from parents about accidents. Where local authorities had pursued cancellation or refusal of registration, they had been 'successful', either in court or in terms of being backed by committee and the provider not appealing, the latter being the most common resolution.

Use of the law represents only the tip of the iceberg in terms of how regulation officers respond to service providers who do not meet the standards required. Officers often said that any threat of refusal was sufficient for potential service providers to withdraw from the process of registration. Officers also described how they had 'counselled people out' of the registration process at an early stage. The more rigorous nature of the standards in the Children Act than those in previous legislation often acted as a deterrent to childminders who were not committed to the role expected of them. Some officers however described cases which they had registered where they had concerns because the grounds for not doing so were not considered sufficiently substantial. Cancellation of registration was considered even more difficult than refusal because counselling out was no longer possible and parents often supported the service provider when legal action was threatened. One officer said:

> *I feel we've lost a few battles with providers we should have won in the early days. Those were people registered by the patch workers [before the Children Act] who didn't really have the clout to get them up to good standards. We could have rectified that when the Children Act came in but we didn't.*

The need for local authorities to make a watertight case based on extensive evidence built up over a period of time was highlighted and the judgement in the Sutton case had, as noted earlier, contributed to a climate of some caution in enforcing the legislation in many authorities. This was also reflected in the number of officers who expressed the need for training in using the law, as noted above. Less than half of the regulation managers in seventeen authorities thought that the Children Act had made it easier to refuse or cancel registration, only one thought it was harder. The rest either did not know or thought there had been no change.

*The view from service providers*

The new national framework of standards and the introduction of the annual inspection duty had potentially profound consequences for providers of day care. At the time of implementation, Guidance suggested that changes to the physical environment, staffing levels and training, and policy, practice and equipment may all be required in order that service providers meet the requirements of the new system. The new duty to inspect services annually created a new framework for an on-going relationship between providers of services and the regulating authority beyond initial registration.

In the first year of implementation, during which time most local authorities focused on the re-registration of services required by the Act, local authorities reported a mixed response to the new regime, with considerable resistance from a significant minority of providers. Anxiety about the exacting nature of the requirements during initial stages of implementation was also widely reported by providers in the case studies and this was fuelled by attention in the media to the stringent nature of the regulations and the potentially disastrous consequences of this for children's services. A significant minority of private day care proprietors articulated their concerns at a political level and an organisation representing some private providers published a survey of their members which highlighted some of the difficulties they had faced (NPDNA, 1993).

It is difficult to assess how far this initial reaction to the new regulation system represented a response to a truly 'over-zealous' approach to regulation among some authorities at the time when the Act was implemented. No evidence of an over-rigid application of standards was apparent among authorities in the study sample in the first year of implementing the Act. Standards applied nearly always conformed exactly to those set out in Guidance; very few higher ratios were applied (see also Ball, 1993). All authorities said that they gave time for service providers to meet requirements made of them.

The service providers survey conducted in summer 1994 offered the first indications of how the new system was working from a providers' perspective at a national level, by which time most providers in England had experienced their first annual inspection visit. It gave a clearer indication of the nature and extent of changes that service providers had been required to make as a result of requirements under the new system. Most providers had made changes to their service as a result. The most common changes for childminders and playgroups were the purchase of new health and safety equipment or to arrangements for record keeping. For day nurseries, they were more likely to involve changes to premises.

Local authorities had, it would appear, adopted an incremental approach to requiring these changes by allowing service providers time to make them in most cases. However, only one-fifth or less of service providers had been offered any financial help to make the changes required of them. This raises the difficult issue of how raising standards in day care can be resourced within an unsubsidised private market of provision. Clearly, if the costs of improving premises, buying new equipment and training staff are passed on to the consumer, services may become unaffordable to all but those with the greatest purchasing power; existing evidence suggests that many families with low incomes have difficulty in meeting even the modest fees currently charged in many playgroups (Statham et al., 1990). Reducing standards in the interests of maintaining levels of provision at low cost is likely to compromise any ambition to promote quality beyond the most basic requirements for safety.

However, despite this tension between regulation, expansion and affordability, less than a quarter of providers from each service type in the service providers survey thought that the new system had stopped them from expanding or developing their service; here, as with the statistical evidence reviewed in chapter 1, there seems little evidence that the implementation of the Children Act affected real growth in provision. Moreover, the principle of regulation was almost unanimously supported by day care providers and the actual experience of inspection in practice had been largely positive. Most service providers thought their local authority's standards were 'about right', but a significant number of day nurseries were less satisfied, describing standards as 'too strict' or 'inconsistent' (figure 4.2). Indeed, overall, the survey results indicate that responses to regulation among providers varied according to service type, with private day nurseries more critical than other providers. One explanation for this would be that it is in the private, for-profit sector, that the tension between meeting standards and keeping costs down is at its most acute.

**Figure 4.2: Attitudes to LA standards**

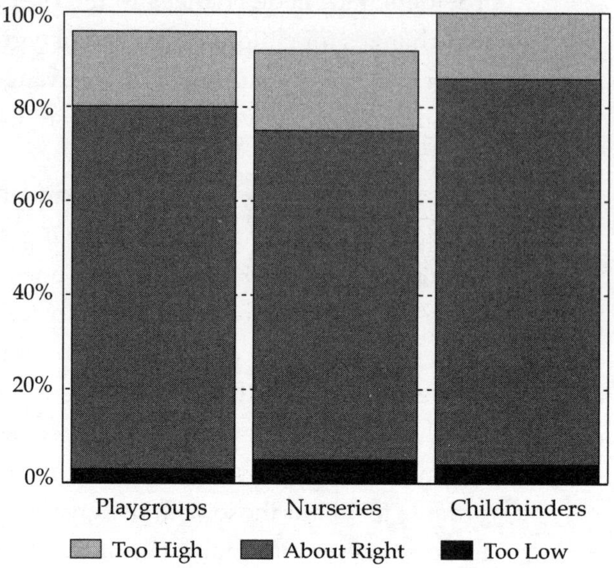


Local context was also an important mediating factor affecting the response of providers to the new regime, as work in the case studies went on to explore in more depth. These case studies revealed how, in practice, the response from service providers was heavily influenced by the nature of the change represented by the new system at a local level, how much this change represented a break from the past, and how this change has been resourced and managed locally. Whether a new regulatory culture (in terms of a change from a developmental and supportive to a more remote style of inspection) had emerged from the implementation of the Children Act, was also important. For example, where service providers had lost the local contact with a day care adviser because of a move to arms length inspection, they often complained of the loss of support this entailed. By contrast, in another authority which had moved only private day nursery inspection into their inspection unit, provider representatives welcomed the change and the perceived increase in professionalism which it was thought to have brought about. It may be therefore that different types of service have different needs in terms of support and different expectations of the regulation system. Another influential factor was likely to be the extent to which providers were involved in developing the local guidelines, including how far they had been consulted about local standards.

Provider organisations, although not asked specifically about registration and inspection, often spontaneously talked of regulation when asked about their relationships with the local authority and the general impact of the Children Act. This, in itself, indicates the importance of the registration process in acting as an interface between the local authority and service providers. Again, many service provider organisations were broadly positive and talked of how the Act had raised standards in the services they represented and improved the nature of their contact with the local authority. Difficulties mentioned included the training requirement and the requirement to keep records on children. One comment found among PLA chairs was that the local authority required changes but offered no resources to fund them, and one chair described how the demands on low-paid workers were increasing because of regulation: 'some workers feel very poorly paid for a job that's become very formal'. In local authorities where there were difficulties with the staffing and management of regulation, problems in the relationships between voluntary sector representatives and the local authority were more likely to be reported.

Within a broad picture of a positive response from providers to regulation, one area stands out as problematic on the basis of data collected in both the service providers survey and the case studies: that of how providers have responded to local authorities' handling of issues of diversity of race, culture and language. For example, a significant minority of providers said that the issue had not been discussed with them by the local authority when they were inspected. A large minority of providers from each type also said that they thought the emphasis placed on the issues by the local authority was 'too much' (figure 4.3).

The survey data add to a picture gleaned through work in the case studies of unease among regulation officers and providers with this new aspect of the regulation system. Registration officers frequently commented that they were unsure of how to put across issues to providers and felt that they themselves needed more training in this area. They reported that providers often failed to see the relevance of the issue particularly in 'white areas' where service providers had no or very few children from minority ethnic backgrounds. The issue of diversity was most often perceived by both officers and service providers as centring on issues of 'race' rather than those of gender or disability.

Incorporating equal opportunities issues into the legislative framework for regulation is challenging because the issues are concerned with attitude and awareness and therefore not easily amenable to a checklist style of assessment. Not surprisingly therefore, training for both officers and

**Figure 4.3: Attitudes to LA emphasis on equal opportunities**

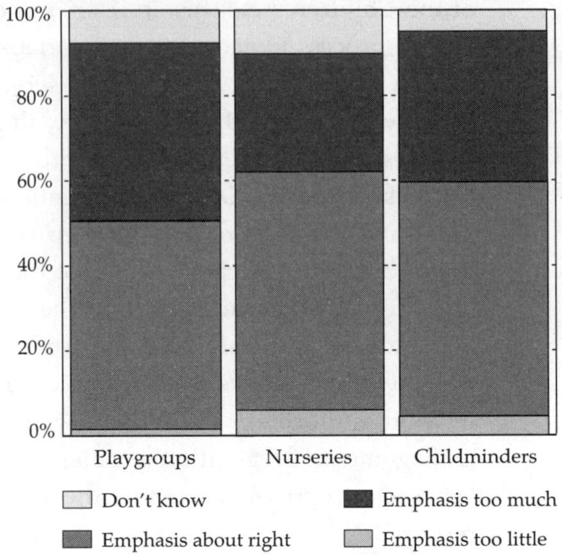


service providers was widely perceived to be needed, as was support for providers making changes to policies and practices to reflect ethnic and cultural diversity. This provided one illustration of the way in which the inspection process raises issues of training and support which require follow-up beyond annual inspection.

**Evaluation of the Act**

*Perceived impact*

The reformed duty to regulate day care services has clearly made a significant impact within local authorities and, in terms of resources, organisational change and direct effects on providers, represents the area where the most change has resulted from Children Act implementation. The new registration and inspection system introduced by the Act is now well established in most local authorities with services re-registered under the new system and most having received their first annual inspection. For most local authorities this has involved considerable reorganisation of staff and a complete overhaul of administrative systems and documentation. In many authorities, the bulk of work involved in implementation of the system is now complete. Among service providers the picture is one which suggests that initial problems which occurred during the transition to the new system have abated as implementation has proceeded, although a significant minority of private day nursery providers remain critical of aspects of the regulatory regime.

The initially positive response to the changes brought by this part of the Act among local authorities remains and is sustained by the widespread view among both managers and officers involved in registering and inspecting services that there have been positive advances among service providers in terms of standards and quality of care achieved. Only four of the 17 managers of registration and inspection services were anything but positive about the impact of the Act, and only five of the 61 officers interviewed thought the impact had been negative or there had been no change. While there is no extensive information by which to judge whether the system appears to be more effective than previous arrangements for registration, most local authority officers report a significant improvement. The following positive outcomes of the Act were repeatedly identified by local authority officers in their overall evaluation of the system:

- raised standards;
- improved status and professionalism of childminders;
- opened dialogue, relationships with providers;
- improved consistency;
- raised awareness about quality, equal opportunities, training;
- standardised procedures.

These responses are very similar to those reported by McQuail and Pugh (1995: 108) in their study of 11 local authorities, in which 'the conclusion of officers across all study authorities was that the registration process is slowly improving, alongside an improvement in standards in services'.

*Differences among local authorities*

There is clearly much variation between authorities in the way in which the regulatory function is delivered. These differences appear in the organisation of the duty (most particularly in how this relates to support), the level of resources dedicated to the task, the approach to the registration and inspection process, and the orientation towards using the law to enforce standards. These differences are not distinct but overlap, so that organisational differences may affect aspects of the registration and inspection process, and the question of resources permeates all areas of the task. For example, an authority which conforms to a greater degree with an 'arms length' approach to inspection is likely to conduct inspection in a different way to those which see it as an on-going developmental process. However, authorities who are committed to combining inspection with support are unlikely to achieve their aims unless they have sufficient staff to undertake additional visits.

The effect of the differences is that local authorities have different regulatory styles with rather different objectives or emphases within a common national framework. These differences are explained in part by the different managerial, organisational and administrative contexts within local authorities, but they also reflect the view held by local authorities of their role in relation to under eights services: whether they see themselves as key providers and funders of services, or as more autonomous enforcers of standards within an otherwise free market of provision. This difference in underlying values will affect where local authorities locate themselves in relation to the model outlined at the beginning of this chapter.

*Issues*

Within these differences, however, some common issues about the regulation of services for young children remain. The first and perhaps most fundamental point is that of how the regulatory task is conceived and defined; that is whether the Act is a framework for ensuring minimum standards of care relating to basic safety requirements or is a tool for promoting quality early learning experiences. The Act and Guidance themselves have always been ambiguous in this respect. Circular LAC (93)1 directs local authorities towards a more minimal approach to regulation, but recent pressures in national policy debates are for registration and inspection procedures to evaluate some elements of the quality of educational experience offered in services, for four year olds, at least. If judgements about the quality of services are implied in the regulation process, and many officers undertaking the task perceive this to be the case, then the basis on which quality is to be assessed is also ill-defined. Moreover, tackling issues related to quality in services, as local authorities have found, raises issues about the need for support and training among providers, which are not easily resolved through regulation alone.

An additional issue is the tension local authorities are attempting to resolve within the regulation role between ensuring a continued supply in the 'mixed economy' of services and ensuring standards/quality of care. In the private sector, the costs associated with complying with standards may force parental fees upwards, in the voluntary sector they may threaten the continued existence of provision. It was just this tension which was addressed by Circular LAC (93)1 which exhorted local authorities to adopt a flexible approach in order to facilitate the goal of expanding services. While the idea of flexibility has been embraced by most local authorities in implementing the Act, some believe it to be at the cost of their ability to enforce standards effectively in all but the most serious of breaches. Moving beyond standards towards quality is equally compromised.

Beyond the policy tensions and ambiguities which underlie this area of the Children Act, there are also practical, managerial and administrative problems which have arisen during implementation. Most obviously there are serious problems with the way the task has been resourced in a significant minority of authorities, and the variations in the workload of regulation staff in authorities with comparable numbers of services remains considerable. This suggests that the rigour of the inspection process is being compromised in some areas, with potentially serious consequences for children. A larger number of authorities are coping with the workload of statutory inspections, but have concerns about the lack of follow-up they are able to do. Adequate numbers of staff are one dimension of implementing the new system effectively, but defining the skills required of staff and training them appropriately are equally important. At present there appears to be no consensus about the 'core skills' required of officers and there is considerable variation in the training they receive.

If we return to the question of the success or failure of the regulatory regime introduced by the Act, we must once again question the original objectives it contained. It is argued here that these were unclear at the outset in terms of the balance to be struck between ensuring standards and promoting quality. Subsequently, they have come into conflict with the broader objective within day care policy of ensuring a supply of services at an affordable cost, within the mixed economy of provision. The balance of powers and responsibilities to be struck between regulators in relation to parental choice and responsibility has been further called into question by the Sutton judgement. Both of these developments contribute to the sense of competing policy objectives and more importantly, of policy objectives which have shifted over time. The question of the relative weight to be given to the welfare of children within these other objectives seems to have become increasingly marginalised. The recent initiative concerning the voucher system adds a new emphasis on learning outcomes to be incorporated into the current inspection regime for children of a certain age in certain types of facility. This will add another dimension to the already diverse range of aims implicit in the current inspection regime.

Given that policy is far from constant and that there is no measure of 'success' in terms of a quantifiable improvement in quality of services, we must be tentative in a judgement about whether the Act has achieved what it set out to do in the area of regulation. However, it is clear that despite some outstanding issues in implementation which have been discussed here, the new regulatory framework has been enthusiastically received and implemented by local authorities as well as being broadly welcomed by providers and their representative organisations. It forms an important part of the interface between service providers and the local authority and despite differences of organisation and style between local authorities, ensures a stronger foundation of minimum standards to protect the safety and well-being of the large numbers of children who attend some form of day care service. It may also, in some cases, provide the platform from which questions about quality can be raised and addressed. As such, it provides an important framework to underpin the diverse range of services provided for young children in Britain today.

**Lessons from the Research**

- Whatever the organisational model adopted by an authority, the exact nature of the support role included in the inspectors' duties should be clear to both officers and providers. Where the support role ends in the inspection process, inspectors should be clear about alternative sources of support and training to which they can refer service providers.

- Large variations in workload within and between authorities are not conducive to consistent practices or equity of treatment for providers. Guidelines are needed at a national level about what constitutes an 'appropriate workload' for an inspector in terms of the numbers of each type of facility which should not be exceeded, in order to help local authorities determine a reasonable level of staff resources.

- Inspectors need good managerial and administrative support to perform their duties effectively.

- Inspectors need training in a range of 'core skills' to perform their role effectively. These skills should be identified so that training can be developed within local authorities, or by using outside trainers.

- The inspection process should encourage a reflexive response from providers which enables them to reflect on their daily practice. A checklist style of inspection format is unlikely to achieve this.

- In order that requirements and recommendations arising from inspection are met by providers, there need to be clear mechanisms for monitoring whether service providers have complied with them. This will entail extra visits, at least to some providers.

- Experiences of refusing and cancelling registration need to be collated and disseminated among authorities with a view to developing guidance on using the law effectively.

CHAPTER

5

# Support for Day Care Services

**Peter Moss**

## Background

Local authorities have, to varying degrees, long provided various kinds of support to private day care providers, both directly and through grant-aiding voluntary organisations. The Children Act, however, recognised this function for the first time in legislation by giving local authorities a specific power to

> *provide facilities (including training, advice, guidance and counselling) for those – (a) caring for children in day care; or (b) who at any time accompany such children while they are in day care (s. 18 (3)).*

Although the term 'support' is not used, section 18 falls within Part III of the Act which refers to 'Local Authority Support for Children and Families'.

It is in the Guidance that the term 'support' is actually attached to this power 'to provide facilities'. The scope and purpose of the power are elaborated in a section headed 'Support Services for Workers and Parents':

> *Section 18(3) gives local authorities power to provide facilities such as training, advice, guidance and counselling to people working in a day care setting (including childminding)...This power is not limited to providing services for people working with or accompanying children in need. It enables local authorities to help people working in day care and childminders raise their standards (DoH, 1991: para. 3.34).*

Guidance therefore enables, but does not require, local authorities to assume some measure of responsibility for general day care services beyond simply their regulation. This role is further emphasised in the approach to regulation recommended in parts of the Guidance with their emphasis on using the regulatory role in a developmental way, to encourage and support services to improve their standards:

> *registration has to be a positive process, there to help the setting up of good quality services...local authorities therefore should use this func-*

*tion in an enabling and facilitating way and seek to encourage developments (ibid.: paras 4.9–4.10)*

*the main purposes of inspection (include)...to encourage day care providers and childminders to raise standards (ibid.: para. 8.7).*

**The Wider Debate**

As already noted in Chapter 4, there has been some debate about the location of regulation in relation to support and development work, with considerable diversity in the solutions local authorities have adopted. Some local authorities have placed regulation in 'arms length' inspection units, others have placed it in mainstream social services departments and others have adopted a split solution. We have shown that there is strong approval among regulation staff for combining support with regulation – although the extent and meaning of the support envisaged varies, a subject returned to later in this chapter.

In considering support, and its importance, three issues need to be borne in mind. First, as we have noted in the Introduction, private day care services for young children are in many ways different to other private services in the welfare system, which are also the subject of regulation. Day care services consist mostly of a large number of individual carers working from home (childminders), and small, part-time non-profit centres (playgroups), who between them account for a workforce of nearly 150,000 workers; while the number of full-time, for-profit businesses (private day nurseries) is growing, they account for less than 5 per cent of all the private day care services that require regulating and may be the subject of support. In short, regulation and support involves working with a large number of very small-scale and geographically dispersed services.

Second, most of the workforce in day care services have a low level of basic training in working with young children. For example, whereas the standard basic training for staff in UK day nurseries is an NNEB qualification or its equivalent, involving a two year post-16 training, in Scandinavia and Spain the basic training for centre-based staff working with children from 0–6 years is at least a three year, post-18 qualification (EC Childcare Network, 1996a). Moreover, the great majority of childminders and playgroup workers in the UK will not even have basic training at a level equivalent to the NNEB.

Third, the demands being made of private day care providers are increasing. Improved regulation has increased the expectations placed on many private providers; but as we have argued in chapter 4, regulation by itself cannot be expected to raise standards. The Children Act encourages local authorities to use private providers for placing children 'in need', with all that means in terms of added requirements to enable providers to respond adequately to the needs of these children. The general increase in the number of children from economically disadvantaged families and the growing instability of family life are also likely to place growing demands on workers in services providing for young children. Last, but not least, the increasing emphasis on day care services having an educational component, at least for children over three (cf. DoH, 1991: para. 6.40 and the proposed voucher scheme to offer education for all four year olds) also presumes an increasingly well-trained workforce.

Finally, it should be noted that the implementation of the Children Act has largely coincided with the introduction of a National Vocational Qualification (NVQ) in 'Childcare and Education'. The NVQ is a competency-based assessment of skills acquired in the workplace. Its introduction provides another example of how the context of day care services has changed, making it harder to attribute change specifically to the Act rather than other factors or the interplay between the Act and these factors.

This new qualification is the subject of much debate. On the one hand it has an extraordinary radical potential, offering the opportunity for women (and occasionally men) to be formally accredited for the skills they have built up over many years of work, paid or unpaid, with children. It can be regarded as a liberating form of qualification, enabling workers to develop self-reflective and critical practice. On the other hand, the level of assessment – 2 or sometimes 3 – is still basic, nowhere approaching the rigour of training required for teaching or social work in this country or for work in services for young children in some other European countries. From this perspective it is a very basic rating of performance, merely enabling those who have completed the assessment to progress to more detailed and rigorous assessment or to enter more formal training. Moreover, while in theory opening up opportunities for a wide range of staff, in practice these opportunities may be denied because the NVQ is not generally eligible for education grants, so the full costs must be borne by the employer or worker herself – unless a local authority or local TEC provides funding – a significant issue given the low pay of many workers in day care services.

**Implementation Three Years after the Act**

*Direct local authority input*

Only three local authorities had staff whose job was *exclusively* to provide support for private day care providers. In one case, this consisted of one part-time Training Officer. In the other two cases, the staffing was rather more substantial, involving the establishment of 'dedicated' support teams. One authority had 8½ full-time equivalent 'Under Eights Development Officers' based on social services area offices. Three-quarters of their time was allocated to development and training, and the remainder to other support; this authority had over 2,200 private providers for children under five (i.e. day nurseries, childminders, playgroups). In the other authority, which had over 3,200 providers, there were 5 full-time equivalent Development Officers, whose remit was to assist voluntary sector organisations, organise training and support small groups such as parent and toddler groups; there were private sector services for children.

All three of these authorities had placed regulation in a separate independent inspection unit, and in all cases the regulation manager interviewed confirmed that regulation staff in these independent inspection units did not have a *formal* support role. This was also the case in two other local authorities with regulatory duties located in independent inspection units, but who had no 'dedicated' support workers. Overall therefore, support was not regarded as a formal part of the regulatory staff's role in a majority of authorities (5/8) with this type of regulation structure, while it was regarded as such in all other local authorities.

However, the view from the ground was not so clear-cut. Even in the five local authorities where the regulation manager said that regulation staff did not have a formal support role, a majority of those officers said that they provided support *informally*, as did the senior regulation officer in one case:

> *You can't run away from the formal role, you can't turn away from advice on the phone. In my view there is a some conflict of interest, but I wouldn't scrap the informal role.*

All authorities had some regulation staff who regarded themselves as having a support role – in fact, only three of the 54 regulation officers interviewed reported that support was not part of their job. The remaining regulation officers divided between a majority who described support as a 'formal' part of their job and a minority, all located in independent inspection units, who said that although not a formal part of their work, they offered some support 'informally'. Put another way, all regulation staff not in independent inspection units said that support was a formal part of their work, compared to a minority of regulation staff in independent inspection units.

Support, however, took second place in the work of staff engaged in regulation. Whether their support role was considered formal or informal, nearly every regulation officer estimated that less than half of their time was allocated to support work, and two-thirds estimated that support accounted for less than a quarter of their work time. Moreover, no local authority had a formula for determining what would be an appropriate level of staffing for support (one had a formula which purported to define staffing levels for regulation and support).

The most common form of support, mentioned by senior officers with responsibility for organising support to providers in nearly all local authorities, was that of visiting service providers experiencing problems, providing training courses and offering telephone advice. Most also offered some general support visits and work on development of new services. Least common, reported in only a third of local authorities, was material support, loans or grants for toys or equipment; this low emphasis on material support was consistent with findings from the service providers survey that less than a fifth of providers required to make changes as a result of re-registration or inspection had received any help with making the change, either in the form of grants or advice (Moss et al., 1995). The training work most frequently mentioned by regulation officers themselves was pre-registration courses for childminders (which in many cases were part of the registration process).

All authorities had an input into training for independent service providers, either through running courses themselves or funding courses run by voluntary organisations or contributions from their staff. Once again, this was mainly for playgroups and childminders. The main direct input (and the most common way in which regulation staff contributed to training) was through pre-registration courses for potential childminders which were universally provided (in most cases directly by local authorities themselves, with the remainder funding others to run them) and post-registration courses (run by half the authorities and funded by a further three). In two cases, education authorities had a direct input into training for private service providers (over and above grant-aiding voluntary organisations): in one case, via an education-based Under Eights Coordinator, who had a small training budget as well as contributing to some pre-registration training for childminders; and in the other via a joint education/social services post, which held a small (£15,000) multi-agency training budget.

Only two authorities had a multi-agency training group and only five had collected information of any kind on the training needs of private day care providers. This was done to varying degrees of thoroughness and in varying ways, as can be seen from the respondents' comments quoted in box 5.1. It is possible that this underestimates the potential availability of information on training needs, since inspection reports may have covered this issue. However, in only one case (quoted in box 5.1) was this source explicitly referred to, suggesting that if the information was sometimes collected as part of inspection it was not necessarily collated and applied as the basis for developing a general training strategy.

**Box 5.1**

**Collection of information on training needs of private providers**

- 'Information is routinely collected by Day Care Advisers via inspection and support visits and responded to...We design and put on training programmes in response to identified needs'.
- 'We canvassed childminders in some parts of the City, for example using the Newsletter to seek childminders' views or when childminders met in groups'.
- 'We sent a questionnaire to childminders in 1993. The aim was to provide a basis for post-registration training...We got 200 replies. First Aid and food hygiene were most popular, how to run a childminders' group was least popular. The training has been postponed to 1995'.
- 'Through the Early Years Forum, which has a sub-group on training'.
- 'Information on needs is collected annually as part of the grant-aiding system'.

*Local authority support for voluntary organisations*

The support outlined so far has focused on that provided directly by local authorities, mainly by their own staff. The use of the power to provide support was however commonly supplemented by making grants to voluntary organisations which also undertook support work with private providers, in particular offering advice and training. Given the limited time available to local authority staff for providing support, the role of voluntary organisations becomes particularly important.

With two exceptions, all local authorities made such grants to voluntary organisations, most commonly to local playgroup and local childminding groups. Most grants came via social services departments but also in some cases through other departments; for example, several education departments made grants to playgroups, but none to childminders. Outside the local authority itself, in five cases TECs were mentioned as giving grants, usually for school-age childcare.

More details on the size and nature of this indirect form of local authority support were provided in the interviews with representatives from voluntary organisations, in particular the local playgroup and childminding groups; all but two of the former and half of the latter got local authority grants. The size of these grants varied considerably: for playgroups from £600 a year to £150,000, and for childminders from £150 to £39,000. However, since the number of providers also varied considerably between local authorities, a better basis for comparison is to consider how grants work out per place (although for playgroup organisations the resultant figure quoted below overestimates resources because the calculation takes no account of parent and toddler groups, for which support workers were often responsible as well as playgroups). For playgroups, the most common level was £5 per place or less a year (9/15), with a further two local authorities granting £6–10 a year and three £15–25. The remaining grant-giving authority paid an average of £183 per place. The main reason for this much higher level of payment was that this authority was the only one to provide a general subsidy to all playgroups in its area via its grant to the local PLA. In the five other cases where local authority grants were partly used to fund playgroups, this took the form of small grants made to selected playgroups, on a 'one off' rather than a recurrent basis (for example, in one case hardship grants of up to £150 were available, while another PLA branch offered help to 'struggling' playgroups in areas of high need). The most common use of local authority grants was to support PLA fieldworkers and training costs (12/15) and the local PLA organisation (rent and other office costs) (11/15).

Childminding organisations were not only less likely to get grants, but also got lower levels of grant, in no case over £6 per place. Where received, however, grants were mainly used to fund local organisations and support work.

Not only were the grants overall at best modest; in a few cases they were positively miserly. The chair of one local childminding group, with 800 members, reported her organisation received £150 a year from the local authority. The group had applied for grants for training, but had been turned down. As a consequence, all training arranged by the group, for example in first aid, had to be self-financing, in other words childminders had to pay themselves. Another authority paid its local PLA branch £600 to fund one fieldworker, a sum reduced from £800 the previous year and in response to a modest application for £1500.

In this case, as others, low grants were stretched by the voluntary organisations receiving them by reliance on low pay and poor employment conditions for their support staff. For example, a £70,000 grant by one large local authority to the local playgroup organisation had to cover not only 'one off' grants to playgroups and support for training, but also the costs of twelve fieldworkers; the chair of the organisation observed that even with a substantial recent increase in grant, the rate of pay for these support workers remained poor. In another large local authority, a grant of £5,000 was only enough to cover the expenses of playgroup support workers, with no salary element. A grant of £32,000 a year in a third authority, again with a large population, had to cover office rent, 'hardship' grants to playgroups and the salary of a training co-ordinator and four fieldworkers, none of whom had received a pay increase over the preceding three years, and each of whom had responsibility for 50 playgroups and 50 parent and toddler groups.

The trade-off between staffing levels and employment conditions was illustrated very clearly by the experience of one local childminding organisation. This organisation had decided to reject low pay scales for support workers. But raising pay levels had only been achieved at the expense of employing one less support worker – and even so, the remaining support workers still only received £3.92 an hour plus expenses, a figure well below average earnings for women workers[4].

4. According to the 1994 New Earnings Survey, average earnings were £7.42 an hour for women employed full-time in non-manual occupations.

Overall, therefore, support work in most local authorities was undertaken by a mixture of local authority staff, who combined the work with regulation, and staff working for voluntary organisations, mainly grant-aided for this purpose by local authorities. In the remaining minority of authorities, there was either a group of 'dedicated' local authority support workers or else no staff with a formal support role. There was no obvious relationship between direct and indirect input by local authorities into support; for example, the two local authorities with no staff with a formal support role did not provide high levels of funding to voluntary organisations to undertake support work.

*The service providers' view*

The results from the service providers' survey indicate that most providers felt there was someone available 'whose job it is to offer you advice or support'. Less than a quarter of providers in each of the three provider groups covered in the survey said they had no-one, the proportion being lowest for childminders and highest for day nurseries. The main people mentioned were local authority staff (either inspection officers or other staff). Playgroups were twice as likely to refer to support from voluntary organisations as day nurseries or childminders. This may reflect not only the well established and geographically widespread support network of the PLA, but also the fact that playgroups were more likely to be members of a voluntary organisation (81 per cent were members of the PLA) than childminders or day nurseries[5].

Not only did many providers see local authorities as the place to go for support; over three-quarters of providers in each group also found 'social services readily accessible by telephone' and most, though slightly fewer, service providers felt they could talk to social services about anything. However, this left a substantial minority who felt either that they could only talk to social services about something serious or could not talk to them at all. Although these reservations were most widely reported by private day nurseries (36 per cent), less so by playgroups and childminders (both 23 per cent), it was day nurseries who were most likely to have contacted their local authority for advice or other support in the 12 months preceding the survey: two-thirds had been in touch for advice or other support, compared to a half of playgroups and just over a third of childminders. While there was little difference between the three groups

5. Day nurseries which belonged to an organisation were much more likely to be members of PLA than of an organisation specifically for private day nurseries, such as PDNA.

in the proportion who had made one contact – around a quarter – there was considerable variation in the proportion who had made contact more than once, ranging from 44 per cent of day nurseries to only 12 per cent of childminders, with playgroups midway between these two extremes. Two-thirds or more of service providers who had contacted their local authority had found the contact helpful, with childminders most positive (82 per cent) and day nurseries least positive (67 per cent).

Overall, therefore, a picture emerges of service providers feeling they have someone in their local authority to contact for advice and other support, quite frequently doing so and finding their contacts generally helpful – but with private day nurseries not only making most contact but expressing rather more reservations than childminders or playgroups. Voluntary organisations are also important, though less so, for support, although service providers were not asked for their views on the accessibility and helpfulness of these organisations. A third potential source of support was also touched on in the service providers survey. About a half of all service providers reported having regular contact with other providers.

Finally, turning from general support for private providers to support for the particular situation of private providers taking children 'in need' placed by local authorities, s. 17(5) of the Act requires local authorities to facilitate provision of services for children 'in need' by private providers. Although not specified, support might be assumed to be one means of facilitating this role for private providers. About half of the day nurseries with whom a child 'in need' had been placed by a social worker or health visitor in the twelve months preceding the service providers survey reported receiving extra help for the child, but only a third of childminders and a quarter of playgroups. Telephone and visiting support were the most common forms of help for day nurseries and childminders (in 50–60 per cent of cases); telephone support was the most common form of help for playgroups (55 per cent), but extra staffing was also frequent (50 per cent, compared to 15 per cent of nurseries), ahead of visiting support (32 per cent).

**Evaluation of the Act**

*Perceived impact*

As we have already seen in chapter 2, policy officers in just over a third of local authorities perceived there to have been increased spending on support and training since the implementation of the Children Act, but this area appeared to have had a much lower priority for increased spending than regulation or provision. Taking a broader view, most senior support workers interviewed thought that support for day care services had improved since the Act. Only two thought it had worsened, leaving two who thought it unchanged and one who felt that support had improved in some respects but worsened in others.

Service providers interviewed in the service provider survey were less convinced there had been improvements, although few said there had been any deterioration in support. For those who had been registered before the Children Act, and were therefore in a position to comment, around two-thirds felt the Act had made no difference to the support they got from the local authority. Among those who did feel there had been a difference, the majority (around a quarter of providers in all three groups) felt that support was now better, leaving a small group (ranging from 5 per cent of childminders to 14 per cent of day nurseries) who felt it to be worse. There was a similar pattern of response for the impact of the Act on support from other organisations, with rather more – about three-quarters – saying it made no difference and hardly any providers reporting they felt it had worsened support.

In general, therefore, the Act was seen as neutral or mildly positive in effect on overall support for private providers. However, most local authority support officers interviewed (10/15, plus 1 'don't know') believed that current staffing levels did not enable them to offer adequate support to private providers. Several referred to the consequence of the support function being only a power, rather than a duty:

> *[Support] has probably got worse. Support is seen as a low priority – edged out by statutory visits.*
>
> *I think it should have been better than it is. But it was put in as a 'can' rather than a 'must', so it got lost.*
>
> *The Act emphasised the need for training, but because it wasn't a requirement, it was a low priority. There is no firm agreement with purchasers that day care training is part of the package – it's not explicitly in the package.*
>
> *I think [the Act made support] even more necessary. Standards are much higher. But unfortunately time and money are not allowing us to do this. We tend to react to situations, that's all we can do, it doesn't allow for a lot of on-going work.*

The Children Act and Guidance have focused attention on the issue of training for day care providers. Looking over the five year period from

1989 to 1993, McQuail and Pugh (1995) concluded that 'the amount of training available to most providers appears to have increased' (p.7) in the 11 local authorities they studied. In our study, there was evidence of increased training availability, for example the general provision of pre-registration courses for prospective childminders. In the service providers survey, rather more than half of the providers registered before the Children Act felt that training opportunities had improved or increased since the Act.

At the same time, the great majority of providers in the survey said that they would like more training, either for themselves or their staff. The proportion was highest for day nurseries (91 per cent) and playgroups (85 per cent), but was also very high among childminders (75 per cent). The most frequently mentioned subject for further training was first aid or health and safety, followed by special needs. Similar, but rather lower, levels of interest were expressed in three other topics – play, child development and child abuse. Least interest was expressed in HIV/AIDS, multi-culturalism, curriculum and working with parents. Among nurseries, staff development and management were more frequently mentioned than among playgroups and day nurseries; indeed, staff development was the most sought after area of training for nurseries, ahead even of first aid and health and safety.

Over half the service providers said they had difficulty in finding or attending training courses – ranging from 58 per cent of childminders up to 72 per cent of day nurseries. The difficulties most often mentioned varied somewhat according to the type of provider. All three groups mentioned the timing of courses and both day nurseries and playgroups mentioned cover to release staff. Otherwise, costs were commonly mentioned by day nurseries, transport by playgroups and lack of childcare by childminders.

On the specific experience of service providers who had taken children 'in need' in the preceding 12 months, the great majority of those who had received extra help to support this work described it as good or adequate (although the childminders were less likely than day nurseries and playgroups to describe the help as 'good' and more likely to describe it as 'adequate', suggesting a possible lower level of satisfaction). Only a small group described what help they had got as 'inadequate'. However, while the help on offer was generally well received as far as it went, a substantial proportion of providers said they would have liked additional help – two-thirds of the nurseries, half the playgroups and a third of the childminders. Overall, the great majority of service providers (from 69 per cent of childminders to 84 per cent of playgroups) noticed no change in the support or training available for taking children 'in need', subsequent to the Children Act. Those who had noticed a change were much more likely to say that more, rather than less, was now available, with childminders twice as likely to say there was more support (28 per cent) than playgroups (15 per cent) or nurseries (13 per cent)

While representatives of playgroup and childminding organisations were not asked if they felt the level of support had changed since the Children Act, they were asked if the amount of grant received from local authorities had changed over the preceding three years, that is, since implementation of the Act. Childminding organisations were less likely to get a grant, and those that did were equally divided between the grant having remained the same and the grant having increased. Nearly all playgroup organisations received some funding, and were nearly equally divided between reporting an increase, no change and a decrease.

The playgroup organisation in one authority had seen an increase in grant from £25,000 to £70,000 in one year (although this higher figure still only worked out at £5 per year per playgroup place because of the large number of playgroups and taking no account of any work undertaken with parent and toddler groups); the organisation was certain that this was due in considerable measure to the Children Act, which 'was a lever, a definite stimulus'. The playgroup organisation in another authority had received an extra £10,100 since 1993, £10,000 for training from education and £100 from social services. Reduced grants might be due, as in one case, to the general financial state of the local authority, while in other cases they were made for reasons not apparent to the organisations:

> *[Over the last 3 years, the playgroup organisation has been] severely cut. Three years ago we got £20,000, now its £10,000.We cannot put on training courses...The reasons for the cuts were not given. The local authority said it did not see the need for a county organisation and disbarred us from applying for funds, so our branches have to apply [on our behalf].*

Finally, one playgroup organisation reported a substantial increase in its direct grant from the education department of its local authority – but had then suffered a large indirect cut due to changes in further education funding; previously, the cost of training courses had been free to PLA members, but this was no longer so as colleges now managed their own funds.

*Issues*

'Support' covers not only a range of activities, but a number of functions. It can also operate at different levels of intensity. This is one reason why the question about whether workers who regulate services should also have a support role is harder to answer than might at first sight appear – or at least why the responses to the question are not always easy to interpret. It is also the reason why, as we shall see below, managers may say that regulation officers have no formal support role, while some of those regulation officers themselves may say that they do.

In practice, support may involve being available to answer questions and to try and provide advice in reaction to providers' queries. This is the most informal level and is perceived as part of their work by most regulation staff even in the most 'arms length' independent inspection unit, not least because it is almost unavoidable in the inspection process itself or in answering the telephone:

> *Support is there, any phone call can be for advice or support, but it's not spelt out in the job description.*
>
> *By being in the childminder's front room, [inspection officers] give advice.*

This informal support may take the form of advising providers where to go for more formal assistance:

> *I would tell them where to go for advice. The informal bit is that you pick up they need it.*

At some point, this 'informal', reactive support becomes more formal and proactive. This may involve making routine visits to providers, to see how they are getting on and encouraging them to raise concerns. Or it may go further still, in which support activities, especially advice and training, become part of a developmental role, concerned actively to raise standards and promote good practice. As already seen in chapter 4, this was often the reason why it was felt that regulation and support should be combined, since they were seen as having a shared objective of raising standards, with regulation providing opportunities for offering support for development. The case studies included several instances of inspection providing a way of setting standards, while support work consisted of encouraging service providers to achieve these standards. For example:

> *An instance of supportive development work, rather than the imposition of requirements, was met in the course of an annual inspection. In this authority, childminders were required to give written responses to questions about their understandings of equal opportunities towards children of minority ethnic groups. The answers given by the childminder the previous year had been judged inadequate, in that she said that equal opportunities practice meant treating all the children the same. The social services worker, who combined development and inspection, had not talked about this with her, at the time. She thought that this would be 'off-putting' and that the childminder's actual work showed a deeper understanding than her answer implied. At the subsequent inspection, however, she brought along some leaflets from the NCMA which explained how treating all children alike was not always appropriate or possible. She left these casually with the childminder as she left, saying she thought she might be interested. She did not remark on the previous year's written answer (Bull et al., 1994b: 26).*

Some regulation officers however made an explicit distinction between 'support' and 'development', sometimes to define the limits of what they felt they should be doing:

> *Support should be limited [for regulation officers] and not combined with development. Support as in advice is appropriate – no-one else does it for the private sector. So regulation officers have a support role but not a development role.*

> *Regulation Officers have a developmental role. As far as time allows, inspection should not be just regulating and monitoring but should allow scope for good practice. A support role implies ready access to talk about anxieties.*

> *The best way to improve quality is to work with providers in a development role over time.*

The most basic issue therefore about support concerns its purpose, and therefore the extent and nature, of support. Support might be seen as a continuum, running from one extreme where local authorities supply limited support to a minority of service providers (e.g. to services in difficulty or to providers taking children 'in need'); through the adoption of a low-level, general developmental role, with programmes of regular visits to providers, grants to voluntary organisations and input to training;

to the other extreme of a high-level, general developmental role, aimed at promoting quality across the board, including grants and other material assistance for services, free or subsidised training and support staff working intensively with small groups of institutions or childminders.

Determining the purpose and level of support is important for several reasons. Most obviously, without clarification of what support is, it is difficult to determine what resources are needed to undertake the work successfully. It is telling that no local authorities in the study had any formula for determining staffing resources needed to undertake support and that, where combined with regulation, support accounted for a minority of the time that regulation staff had available. Even in those two authorities which employed a team of 'dedicated' support workers, the workload for each development worker based on total service providers was, on paper, very large – 250 services per worker in one case, 640 in the other (both excluding any work with services other than playgroups, nurseries and childminding). In local authorities without any dedicated staff, the problem is more acute if only because for the staff combining regulation and support work (whether formal or informal), the support power is in competition for staff time and other resources with the regulatory duty.

Resources are critical, in particular if support is defined as promoting the development of services. This may well involve improvements in accommodation, equipment and other material resources. It will almost certainly involve staff development, in particular improved basic and continuous training given the circumstances outlined in the introduction to this chapter – the low level of training that exists in most UK day care settings, combined with the increasing demands that are being made on staff.

A European example can help to give some indication of what a high level commitment to service development through continuous training might involve. Staff in publicly-funded nurseries in Italy, which are mainly also managed by local authorities, work a 36 hour week of which six hours a week is allocated for contacts with parents and development work such as continuous training and planning work. Service development also involves, in a number of regions, the employment of *coordinatori pedagogici* (pedagogical co-ordinators), support workers who usually have a degree-level training in psychology or pedagogics, and work with a small group of nurseries and nursery schools (around five or six units) to plan and organise continuous training for staff, as well as developing other projects to improve quality and acting as a link between services, the local community and research institutions. Working through these pedagogical co-ordinators, regional and local authorities organise programmes of continuous training for staff (EC Childcare Network, 1996a, 1996b).

Unlike Italy, most UK day care services are privately managed and non-subsidised. In this context, where can or should the resources come from to support and develop these services? The logic of an unsubsidised market, which is the basis of current public policy on day care services, suggests that, as businesses, these costs should be shared between the providers and consumers, except for any general public programmes for business promotion such as those operated by TECs. It is hard to justify social services departments, with their priority to provide for children 'in need', subsidising the development of general services which are deemed to be the private responsibility of parents to pay for and which in some cases (for example, day nurseries) are most likely to be used by higher income families; indeed, it could be argued that it would be more consistent to make support a duty, but link and limit it to the wider duty to provide day care services for children 'in need'.

As with regulation, there appears to be a contradiction between a policy that relies on the one hand on unsubsidised markets and private contracts for the supply of services and on the other hand on public involvement to 'raise standards' in those services, rather than simply ensuring that certain minimum requirements related to health and safety are met. Here, as in regulation, there appears to be a fundamental ambivalence in the Act between private and public responsibility for day care services. The end result is that there is some public investment in support, which has undoubtedly had beneficial results given the low level of service development in general – but this public investment may well prove insufficient either to enforce or to promote voluntarily significantly higher standards across the board. In short, the position of support for day care services as defined by the Act is inherently ambivalent and weak within the broader policy context.

This discussion raises two critical sets of questions. The first arises from the need to define the concept of support from public welfare authorities (either directly or by using public money to fund private organisations to deliver support), and in the light of that how best it should be implemented. What is the purpose of support, particularly in relationship to policy on the supply of services? Who should pay for it? How should it be delivered? Should it be a power or a duty? To answer this set of questions would almost certainly require a broader review of the central component of support, training both basic and continuous, to decide what levels of training would be appropriate to fulfil the social, cultural and educational functions of day care services.

Second, assuming the maintenance of a separate system of 'day care' services, with a strong emphasis on a market model for supply of services, should all services be treated equally with respect to support? Or should a distinction be made between day care businesses (or perhaps businesses of more than a certain size), mainly private day nurseries, and smaller-scale services run either on a non-profit or self-employment basis, mainly playgroups and childminders? The former might be left to respond to market forces, and fund their own development costs, leaving public authorities to focus support work on the latter, possibly using for this purpose a separate and earmarked development fund. To propose this is *not* to accept that the current system is the only way of supplying services; there are alternatives, for example the development of a publicly-funded system of 'services for young children' based on the integration of 'day care' and 'education' services, and such an alternative would have implications for support and development. Rather it is to suggest that the contradictions within the existing system need to be addressed to bring greater clarity to the objectives of support.

**Lessons from the Research**

- As already noted in chapter 2, day care providers need support and training to enable them to offer an appropriate service to children 'in need' Consideration should therefore be given as to whether a duty should be placed on local authorities to ensure appropriate support for all private providers who offer a service for children 'in need' placed with them by local authorities.

- More generally, the support role of public authorities with respect to private providers who are not taking children 'in need' requires clarification. Within this context, the role of different local authority staff and voluntary organisations needs to be clarified for the staff and organisations themselves as well as providers, including the support role included in the duties of regulation officers.

- The skills needed for workers undertaking a support role need to be more clearly identified, so that training can be developed for them.

- Within the context of clarifying the support role, guidelines are needed at a national level about what constitutes appropriate resources for support, covering both local authorities and voluntary organisations, and related to levels of provision and appropriate levels of training, pay and employment conditions for support staff.

- Given the rapid expansion of services, and the fact that staffing across day care services was not reviewed when the Children Act was implemented, nor indeed has ever been, a review of training for workers in day care services (or more broadly in services for young children), both basic and continuous, would be timely.
- The question of access to training, especially for private providers, needs to be kept under continuous review and attention paid to identifying and seeking ways to remove or reduce some of the most common obstacles to accessing training, for example timing, costs and cover.

CHAPTER
# 6 Parents' Perspectives

**Charlie Owen**

## Background

Both the Children Act and its Guidance have very little to say about parents when it comes to day care for under eights. However, the chapter in the Guidance which deals with the section 19 Review of day care does emphasise the need to consult with parents – amongst others – in producing the Review, with a view to working out 'the level, pattern and range of day care and related services for young children' (para. 9.1: see box 6.1).

**Box 6.1**

**Extracts from *Guidance*** [emphasis added]

9.1 The review duty in section 19 gives legislative support to Government policy that the level, pattern and range of day care and related services for young children should be worked out at the local level by local authorities in consultation with health authorities, voluntary organisations, employer interests, *parents* and other interested bodies and individuals....

- effective working relationships should be established and maintained with ... [amongst others], voluntary organisations, the private sector and *parents*.

9.7 Section 19(7) requires the two authorities [*i.e.* local authority and local education authority] to 'have regard to representations from health authorities and any other representations which they consider relevant'...The review should be an open process and early involvement is recommended with the health authorities, voluntary bodies such as local PPA groups, childminding interests, community groups, lone parent organisations and ethnic minority groups, with the private day care sector, employers and *parents*.

9.15 The two authorities should work out their consultation procedures in the light of local circumstances. ... Attention should be paid to ways of seeking views from a cross-section of the population.

**The Wider Debate**

There have been two large scale national surveys of parental preferences with regard to day care. In 1975 OPCS conducted a survey of parents' needs for day care on behalf of the DHSS (Bone, 1977) and a similar survey was conducted by OPCS for the DoH in 1990 (Meltzer, 1994). In these surveys parents were asked both, which services they actually used for their children and what were their preferences. The 1975 survey asked only about under fives but the 1990 survey included children up to eight. It also included questions about informal care arrangements, by unpaid relatives, friends or neighbours. An important feature of these surveys is that they included non-users of services, as these are a much harder group to contact – as local authorities have discovered.

**Table 6.1: Percentage of parents choosing each form of day care as ideal: pre-school children**

| Day care service | Age of child last birthday | | | | | |
|---|---|---|---|---|---|---|
| | 0 | 1 | 2 | 3 | 4 | All pre-school children |
| | Percentage of parents choosing as ideal | | | | | |
| Daily paid help | 17 | 14 | 8 | 10 | 6 | 11 |
| Childminder | 11 | 9 | 9 | 6 | 5 | 8 |
| Day nursery | 6 | 16 | 22 | 18 | 14 | 16 |
| Creche | 21 | 23 | 20 | 15 | 14 | 19 |
| Playgroup | 2 | 14 | 34 | 27 | 22 | 20 |
| Mother and toddler group | 21 | 39 | 22 | 6 | 2 | 19 |
| Nursery school or class | 1 | 5 | 24 | 56 | 68 | 28 |
| None of these | 36 | 13 | 7 | 2 | 3 | 12 |
| Base: | 626 | 739 | 713 | 685 | 475 | 3238 |

Percentages may add to more than 100 because parents could choose more than one form

*Source:* Re-analysis of data from Meltzer (1994).

The 1990 survey included 3,705 households with a child under eight, with 5,525 children overall, including 3,243 under fives who had not yet started school. Meltzer found that, taking all pre-school children together, 6 per cent went to registered childminders, 8 per cent to day nurseries or creches, 15 per cent to nursery schools or classes and 21 per cent to playgroups. In addition, 7 per cent were already attending primary school (33 per cent of four year olds). (Some children attended more than one type of day care.) Most parents expressed considerable satisfaction with whatever service they were using.

However, when asked what they thought was the ideal arrangement for someone of their child's age, parents often chose a different arrangement. As table 6.1 shows, the ideal arrangement varied by the age of the child. For children under one the most chosen option (36 per cent) was no formal day care, with mothers preferring instead to stay with the infants themselves or to use some informal care, such as a relative or friend. Nevertheless, 21 per cent felt a mother and toddler group was ideal even at that age. For children aged one, a mother and toddler group was the option most chosen as ideal (39 per cent); for two year olds it was a playgroup (34 per cent). For older children a nursery school or class was thought most suitable (56 per cent of three year olds and 68 per cent of four year olds), being chosen twice as often as a playgroup for three year olds and three times as often for four year olds. Day nurseries were not the most chosen ideal option at any age, but they were chosen more consistently across the age groups than any other form of care: overall the mothers of 16 per cent of pre-school children included a day nursery among their ideal choices.

These ideal choices were made without any constraints due to availability or cost. Yet these two factors exert an enormous influence on the actual day care choices parents can make. The annual statistics on day care places published by the DoH and those on pre-school education published by the DfEE show that provision is very unevenly distributed across local authorities, and locally is likely to be even more so. Owen and Moss (1989) have looked at geographical variation in the availability of different forms of pre-school day care and education. They found enormous variability in levels of provision for the different services, and the situation has changed very little in the intervening years. Despite a growth in independent day nursery places, these have tended to be in areas that already had more day nurseries.

**Table 6.2: Some examples of consultation strategies**

| Type | Definition | Advantages | Disadvantages |
|---|---|---|---|
| Focus groups | Small, selected groups; a facilitator poses questions to focus discussion; open-ended discussion | Opportunity to present views, to hear from other people and to discuss | Few people involved; unlikely to involve policy makers |
| Meetings – formal | A meeting is called at a specified time and place | Possibility of dialogue with policy makers; can hear the views of other people | Unattractive; intimidating; inconvenient; few people attend; misses non-users |
| Meetings – informal | People invited to meet (singly or in groups) during some other event | Convenient; unintimidating | Unlikely to involve policy makers; may not hear other people's views |
| 'Market research' | Interviewer waits in some public place and approaches likely respondents; usually pre-coded questionnaire | Depending on site, can interview a lot of people quickly; includes non-users | People may be reluctant to talk in a public place; depending on site, may be non-representative |
| Survey | Precoded questionnaire given to selected respondents | Representative samples; includes non-users; can get large numbers | Difficulty in identifying respondents; sometimes low response rates |

So one constraint on parental choice is the availability of services. Another is cost. The Policy Studies Institute (PSI) and the DSS carried out a postal survey of 14,500 Child Benefit recipients on the cost of child care (Marsh and McKay, 1993). The survey covered all ages of children. They found that the parents of under fives were more likely to use professional child care than parents of older children, and to pay much more relative to their own earnings: 'Unavoidably, younger children were more expensive; those paying for pre-schoolers paid £36.60 a week [cf. £20.70 for children 5-10], even though most worked part-time' (ibid., p. 368). These surveys give the general picture of parental preferences, but we were also interested in how local authorities went about consulting parents locally, and what the lessons were from those consultations.

**Implementation**

We wrote to all local authorities in England early in 1995, to ask if they had conducted any surveys of parental perspectives on day care, pre-school education and out of school facilities. We asked for results from any surveys of parental experience or preferences. The aim was to collate the results from a range of surveys to give an overview of parental views. It turned out not to be possible to get any such overview.

Of the 108 local authorities to whom we wrote, 75 replied. Of those, few had conducted any systematic survey of parental views: 47 said explicitly that they had not surveyed parental views. However, many of these said that they had tried to gauge parental views by other means, for example by consultation meetings with parents. One metropolitan authority had distributed questionnaires at these meetings and had more than 1,000 returned, although they supplied us with no actual results. Three authorities said that inspectors distributed questionnaires during their inspection visits to day care services: although the inspectors used the information themselves, none had collated the results to give a more general view. An inner London authority had left questionnaires in public places, such as libraries, but gave no idea of how many were returned, nor any tables of results. One County Council interviewed 11 focus groups of parents, about 70 in all (see table 6.2); a TEC also convened focus groups of parents from six London boroughs, covering children of all ages. In neither case were there any statistical results. One outer London borough interviewed 211 parents of under fives in a shopping centre, but no tables were supplied.

An inner London borough said they had commissioned a survey, but that it had not been approved for release to the public, so no results were supplied. Three local authorities had collected information from the parents of under fives as part of their monitoring of users of social services: one County Council had used MORI to interview parents who had contacted Social Services, and got 32 replies from parents of under fives, whereas another had distributed 18,000 service user questionnaires. That authority had received 683 replies from parents of under fives, and the results were used in their first Review. Six authorities reported that local surveys had been conducted within their areas, four of which were conducted by local universities, including two student projects. All of these were small scale, and in no case were any results supplied. One County Council used Health Visitors to fill in questionnaires with parents when they visited at

39 months. They got 271 replies, and these were collated. Another authority gave questionnaires to parents of children in reception class, asking about their use of services before their children had started. They got 240 replies. Both these methods collected data from representative samples of parents, including those who were not using any day care service.

Overall, the attempt to get a picture of parental perspectives on day care and pre-school education by collating local surveys was a failure. Although most authorities had attempted to consult parents, very few had conducted any systematic survey. Almost none presented any statistical data, and certainly too few for any representative analysis. Nevertheless, many local authorities recognised that they were not doing enough to consult parents and wanted to do better in future. A wide variety of strategies had been employed, and these may well be more appropriate to local needs than a survey. Before commenting on the effectiveness of the different methods, I want to examine what the varied consultations did say about parental perspectives.

*Section 19 Review*

Peter Elfer, of the National Children's Bureau, conducted a thorough analysis of the first Section 19 Reviews for what they said on consultation with parents and parents' views. This analysis was conducted on behalf of the DfE. Elfer reported that, on the basis of the available Reviews, 'every authority has provided some opportunity for the views of parents to be recorded' (Elfer, 1994, p. 2). He divided the approaches into three broad types:

- local authorities that have consulted via a *written document;*
- local authorities that have arranged for *face to face meetings with parents;*
- local authorities that have conducted *formal surveys of parents* (ibid., pp. 2-3).

Elfer put at least 19 in this last category. His definition of a survey was more inclusive than the one used in this chapter; for example, he included the three authorities where inspectors issued questionnaires to parents, but where results were not collated systematically.

Elfer summarised the results of the different forms of consultation under six headings:

- the need for more provision;
- the need for provision that will promote the educational and social development of children;
- the need for reliable standards;
- fees: 'Many parents expressed anxieties about the cost of services';
- services that were geographically accessible;
- views from parents from black and minority ethnic communities (ibid., pp. 6-7).

The first two echo the results of the national survey conducted by OPCS. Meltzer (1994) reported much higher levels of demand for services than actual use, and Elfer says that, 'even in relatively well resourced areas, demand far exceeds supply' (Elfer, 1994, p. 5). As in the OPCS survey, Elfer found a strong wish from parents for more nursery education, although he does go on to say that 'many parents spoke of wanting more day care through day nursery provision because it offered care for younger children than nursery education would, and for longer hours' (ibid., p. 5). This finding is also consistent with the OPCS survey. The parental concern over fees echoes the findings of Marsh and McKay (1993) that formal day care for pre-school children was expensive, and consumed a disproportionate amount of parental income.

**Evaluation of the Act**

The problem for local authorities in consulting with parents is that the exercise might unreasonably raise expectations that services will be provided. In other words, to consult about 'the level, pattern and range of day care and related services for young children' might lead parents to believe that their preferences can be translated into provision. Yet while local authorities were given a duty to consult parents in general, they were given no accompanying duty to provide (except for the minority of children 'in need') nor any extra resources to do so. Local authorities also have 'duties under Part III to facilitate provision of services by other organisations including voluntary bodies and the private sector' (Guidance, 3.4), but, again, no extra resources.

The main demands of parents are now well established, by both the national surveys and local consultation: parents want more nursery education, more day nurseries because of their longer hours and less expensive day care. Any local survey is unlikely to find anything different from this general picture. So what is the role of local consultation?

There are at least two roles for local consultation: one is to monitor change over time, for example to see if preferences change or if overall satisfaction is increasing. The other is in assessing specific local needs. Local situations have specific needs beyond the general issues noted above. These might include issues such as where a new facility should be sited; opening hours; policy on age of entry into school; the representation of cultural diversity, etc. These are all issues that can be addressed locally. They may also be issues not best addressed by a survey: the problem with a survey is that there is no dialogue, no discussion. This is best achieved by face to face contact with parents, and local authorities were very creative in arranging ways of establishing such contact. For example, by organising a Fun Day with events for children and using the opportunity to talk to parents; similarly making use of a Play Bus; or setting up a stall in a shopping centre. One metropolitan authority organised a phone-in. (Examples taken from Elfer, 1994.) Traditional meetings, organised at a fixed time, were much less successful, generally with a very low attendance. Meetings, or more informal discussions, during the session of a nursery, for example, were more successful. However, such meetings would miss non-users of the service. Good practice on consultation needs to be shared more widely, with the more innovative methods being disseminated more extensively.

There is still a role for surveys: they are good for getting simple answers to simple questions, but not for exploring complex issues. If they are repeated, surveys are also a good way of monitoring change over time. However, to be useful some considerable care needs to be taken in preparing and administering a survey. One of the most important considerations is the representativeness of the sample, because if the respondents are not typical of parents in the area then the results can be misleading. Leaving questionnaires in libraries of in social services offices, for example, is not going to get a representative sample. Nor is distributing questionnaires to service users, as that misses out on non-users. Large numbers are not a substitute for representativeness. However, getting a representative sample can be very complex, and might well be something on which local authorities might be given some guidance.

If local authorities are to conduct surveys then some co-ordination between them and the use of some common questions would be most helpful. In this way a national picture could be obtained without the expense of a centralised survey.

**Lessons from the Research**

- Both national and local surveys of parental views have shown that parents want more nursery education, more day nurseries, longer hours (especially for playgroups) and less expensive day care.
- Most local authorities made some attempt to consult with parents, but the consultations were often unsystematic: few conducted surveys of parents.
- A wide range of strategies was adopted by local authorities to get information from parents. Good practice and innovative approaches need wider dissemination.
- If local authorities are to conduct surveys they need to be careful about obtaining representative samples and including non-users of services. There should be some guidance and co-ordination of local surveys.

CHAPTER
7

# Conclusions Hindsight and Foresight

**Peter Moss and Mano Candappa**

In previous chapters we have reported results from a major study of the operation of the Children Act in the area of day care services for children aged under eight, in particular examining its workings and impact three years after implementation. Our main findings are summarised in the Executive Summary at the front of the book, and each chapter has concluded with a number of 'lessons from the research'. But although we have organised the book under a number of specific themes (provision, co-ordination, regulation, support), in practice a number of issues have arisen from the study which cut across these themes. We begin this final chapter by considering some of these 'cross-cutting' issues, before moving on to weigh up the Act, which is now five years in operation, and looking forward to the next five years.

## Cross-cutting issues

- **Resources**: in present circumstances, it is impossible to get comprehensive and reliable information on the total amount of public resources allocated to day care services – or indeed to the whole range of services for young children. Indicators that exist (e.g., staffing and workload levels, provision) suggest that resource allocation is very variable between local authorities and, at least for provision and support, low. Any increased resources allocated by local authorities to services for children under eight since the Act have mainly gone into regulation, although even in this area there remains a wide variation between workload levels in different authorities reflecting different levels of resourcing. Elsewhere, while there are examples of additional expenditure, these are generally modest, and have been offset in some cases by budget cuts.

  What makes the resource issue particularly acute is a history, that long precedes the Children Act, of low overall levels of private and public investment in day care services. This history is reflected today in poor training and pay for many workers in day care services and low levels of publicly funded provision. With this legacy and without a major injection of resources, which seems not to have occurred, the impact of the Act has inevitably been constrained.

- **Expectations on the private and voluntary sectors**: the Act and accompanying Guidance have accorded a central role to the private and voluntary sectors – as service providers, as the subjects of regulation and as partners in the development of services. This was inevitable and necessary given the dominance of these sectors in the provision of day care services (public provision accounts for less than 5 per cent of day care places).

  In general, the voluntary and private sectors have responded very positively to the high profile given to their role. More attention, however, may need to be given to the conditions required to enable the voluntary and private sectors to play their role, fully and effectively. If, for example, the private and voluntary sectors are to play a significant part in providing day care for children 'in need' – and they appear to offer a largely untapped but willing reservoir of providers – this will need to be accompanied by a substantial input of resources to ensure they can be offered appropriate support for meeting the needs of these children and their families. Similarly, if organisations representing providers are to play an active role in providing support for individual providers and in contributing to a co-ordinated approach to the development of services, then not only will they need adequate resources to do so, but they also need to be actively and fully included in coordinating structures and processes. At present, there is a danger of raising expectations about the role of the voluntary and private sectors without providing the means to enable them to fulfil this role adequately.

- **Information**: a recurrent issue in the study has been the inadequacy of information. There is an absence of information systems to supply local authorities, on a regular and reliable basis, with reliable data about need and demand for services, about the services themselves including their usage, staffing and costs, about their regulation and support and about the resources allocated to these services. This is replicated at national level, where the annual DoH returns provide a narrow range of information, essentially a count of places in local authority-run and private services, which in turn are not comparable with the equally narrow range of information on education for children under five produced by DfEE.

This issue is also emphasised by McQuail and Pugh (1995: 3, 118) who in their study of 11 local authorities note:

> *The inadequacy of statistical information on the services young children use. There is a lack of comparability between figures collected by the Department of Health and Department for Education and many categories of provision are either not distinguished in the figures or are not counted at all...A further difficulty was the lack of detailed information [in local authorities] about inputs, outcomes and evaluation of the quality of services.*

- **Diversity**: the Children Act placed considerable emphasis on the need to recognise and respond appropriately to diversity, in particular ethnic diversity, diversity in provision, and disability. The Act has undoubtedly led to greater attention being paid to these aspects of diversity, although there have been some difficulties in giving effect to increased commitment, seen for example in the limited success of local authorities in including minority ethnic groups in the Review process, the doubts expressed by some service providers as to the relevance of addressing issues of ethnic diversity and the marginalisation felt by some voluntary organisations in their dealings with local authorities.

  These dimensions of diversity are however now clearly on the agenda. Others are not, partly because they receive little or no attention in the Act or Guidance, perhaps most notably gender and the material circumstances of families. Diversity can also be considered at an area level, as well as at an individual or family level, for example the different needs and circumstances of urban and rural areas or of areas with high levels of social and economic disadvantage. The great majority of authorities, however, have adopted an individual rather than area-based approach to need, and there were strong forces, in particular resources, supporting this approach.

- **The pre-Children Act inheritance**: as noted in the Introduction and illustrated throughout the study, local authorities started at very different points in their implementation of the Children Act, in terms in resources, provision, policy, structures and, underpinning all of these, priority attached to early childhood services. One group of authorities, in particular, had relatively high levels of publicly funded provision, explicit aspirations to provide a service to all children and an achieved or aspired objective of integrating early childhood services within a single system. In particular, for these authorities the

Children Act has had less significance, not even necessarily raising the profile of services for young children, a benefit quoted in many other cases, since in these authorities services for young children already had an above-average profile.

- **Marginalisation and division of services for young children**: historically, services for young children have had a low priority, both in policy and service terms. There are several contributory causes. Until recently, the UK has had a low level of employment among women with young children, and many mothers who were employed have taken responsibility for managing the relationship between employment and family life by working short hours, often during weekends or evenings, and using informal care arrangements; this has reduced labour market pressures to develop services, which in other countries have been a powerful influence. Public involvement by welfare authorities in the provision of day care services has always been confined to a relatively small group of children defined as 'in need' on narrow welfare criteria, rather than as in many other European countries also supporting employed parents. An early compulsory school age, by European standards, combined with increasing numbers of four year olds starting primary school, has removed another source of pressure for developing services for young children; rather than the development of a separate and substantial pre-primary education stage (as in much of the rest of Europe where the prevailing model is three years pre-primary education from three to six years), nursery education has developed on a very limited scale (part-time and for three terms where it does exist), and following a model (the nursery class attached to a primary school) which reduces its significance.[6]

  These factors, making for the marginalisation of services for young children, have been compounded by the division of responsibility for services for young children between the education and welfare systems. One consequence is that an already low priority area has been split, so becoming even less significant in each of two large systems. This has occurred both at local level and nationally, where early years forms a small part of the organisation of both the DoH and the DfEE.

  One major consequence of the marginalisation and division of services is that early childhood services – whether in welfare or education – are at permanent risk of becoming marginal players in others'

6. For a full review of early childhood services in the European Union, see EC Childcare Network (1996a).

games. Instead of developing a strong, integrated and coherent 'services for young children' agenda, 'day care' services become an item on the welfare agenda of children 'in need' or on the employment and training agenda of labour supply, while nursery education increasingly becomes an adjunct to primary schooling and the National Curriculum. This absorption into other agendas further reinforces the split between day care and education services and further marginalises them within their respective, separate service systems.

Marginalisation and division of services for young children have reduced the impact of the Act on them. Despite the encouragement in Guidance for local authorities to assume a corporate approach to implementation of the Act, in practice (at least in the early years field) it has been regarded as welfare legislation and primarily the concern of welfare authorities (except for the section 19 Review, where the Act places a duty on local education as well as welfare authorities). In particular, education authorities and educational services for children aged under five have had their own agendas and concerns, not to mention a very different culture and mission to welfare. The most serious attempts to grapple with the division of services for young children between the education and welfare systems have resulted not from the Act but from individual local authorities who have sought to integrate responsibility for day care and early years education services, and have done so independently of the Act.

Not only have these structural differences inhibited the Act's ability to promote coordination, but education services for children aged under five have continued to evolve at local authority level very largely independent of day care services and the Children Act; between 1991 and 1994, the number of children under five in publicly funded nursery schooling rose by 8 per cent and in reception classes by 15 per cent. The main expansion of publicly funded general provision has therefore resulted not from the powers given to local authorities in the Act, but from the continuing expansion of early years education by local education authorities, undertaken with little or no reference to the Children Act or day care services. The consequence has been a relatively large public investment in a service (nursery classes, offering predominantly part-time provision for just three terms) with an exclusively educational remit and a limited contribution to make in the provision of either care or family support. In short, the Act has not provided a strong enough framework to actively promote a coordinated approach to the development of publicly-funded services, and in so doing overcome the natural tendency of the divided system to produce services that are limited in scope.

In this context, the proposed vouchers' scheme can be seen as supporting a more co-ordinated approach to the extent that it applies not only to school-based services but also to qualifying 'day care' services; it has recognised that education can and should take place across the range of early childhood services and not just in school-based services in the education system. Yet conceptually, in its emphasis on the education function while ignoring the care and support functions of early childhood services, and organisationally, by locating the initiative in the DfEE, the voucher scheme assumes and reinforces a divided approach to 'early childhood services', reflected in the dual system of inspection that will now apply to 'day care' services which seek eligibility for vouchers.

**Weighing up the Act**

There are many factors which make it difficult to arrive at a precise evaluation of the impact of the Children Act on day care services for children under eight. There is a serious lack of necessary information: for example, base-line data showing how matters stood before the Act (e.g., standards in services), as well as management data for a wide range of post-Act activities. Local authorities were at very different points at the time the Act was implemented, not least in the priority they had previously given to services for young children and the way in which they conceptualised these services. Service development has been influenced by many factors quite external to the Act: for example employment trends and government initiatives emanating from Departments other than the DoH. Overall, any evaluation of the Act as it has affected day care services for young children can do little more than aspire to a broad weighing up, drawing on the more detailed conclusions presented in the earlier chapters.

The Children Act has led to a number of improvements in day care services for children under eight. Overall, they have gained a higher recognition and profile within local authorities. Through the mechanism of the section 19 Review, most authorities now have more information about day care services, both what is available and what is needed. The Act has encouraged a process of better communication and closer working between local authority departments and between local authorities and the private sector, with the section 19 Review again playing an important role. Regulation of services has been overhauled and broadened, bringing with it improvements not only in the regulatory process itself but also, probably, in standards. The welfare role of day care services for severely disadvantaged and distressed children and families has been reinforced and integrated into a wider model of welfare provision, the concept of children 'in need', and the development of innovative approaches to this task has been encouraged. An impetus has been given to addressing the issue of ethnic diversity and how to respond to it in an appropriate way, through the Act and Guidance's explicit recognition of the issue.

These improvements have undoubtedly been worthwhile. They are, however, modest and incremental in nature. A similar conclusion – pointing to real, worthwhile, but limited effect – has been expressed by the Early Childhood Unit at the National Children's Bureau, in its evaluation of section 19 Reviews:

> *Ensuring that the ever increasing diversity of services fits what children and parents need makes a planning and coordinating role imperative. The Review is essential to that role and a stimulus and rationale for debate across all sectors about the quality of experiences offered to children. It is also an essential mechanism to enable parents and children, as users of services, to have a say in their development locally. But guidance on the Review suggests it provides the opportunity for local communities and interest groups to address some of the policy questions facing early years services, that is, how much provision, cost, quality and the balance between universal services and services targeted at families in need.*
>
> *The Reviews cannot determine at the local level these major national policy issues. Rather, national policy, whatever its strengths and weaknesses, will have a major bearing on the shape and conduct of the Reviews by effectively setting their context. If a national policy does not address some of the conceptual differences, or fault lines, that run through our services, two key ones being welfare or education, market or national standards, the Review certainly cannot address them or overcome the tensions they produce in local services (Elfer and McQuail, 1996: 101–102).*

Given the nature of the Act, in relation to services for young children, its limited impact is not surprising. As we argued in Chapter 1, the Act was essentially conservative, building on and tidying up existing policy; it was innovatory in detail rather than principle or approach. With respect to day care services, and in marked contrast to other parts, the Act was based neither on an analysis of existing services, nor any review of past policy and future policy options. The validity and desirability of the welfare/education, 'day care'/'nursery education' split was never considered. A 'co-ordination' model was assumed, rather than tested against an 'integrated' service model. No consideration was given to the issue of the appropriate sharing of responsibility between parents and government for 'day care' services, including the central question of how the cost of services should be allocated. The belief that day care services should be a private responsibility and subject to market solutions, except in the case of children 'in need', was not subjected to scrutiny, nor were the implications for regulation and support of having such a dispersed, small-scale and under-developed supply of private day care.

The Act therefore did not proceed from any broad consideration of general early childhood issues nor from the resolution of a number of important policy questions of an essentially national nature. Nor did the 'day care' parts of the Act benefit from the application of any general 'child welfare' principles, for example the 'paramountcy' principle that the child's welfare is paramount in decision-making. Consequently, the Act's impact on services for young children was bound to be limited.

However, by not addressing some long-standing issues in early childhood services, seeking instead for an improvement of the existing policy approach, the Act in some respects has increased or brought into sharper focus the contradictions already existing in that approach. Is it possible to reconcile a provision policy based on private market principles and sole parental responsibility with an active policy of public regulation, through which Guidance aspires not only to secure minimum standards but also to raise standards? How far can co-ordination between 'day care' and 'education' for young children be promoted by legislation that assumes and reinforces the separateness of 'day care' and 'education' services and is itself firmly located in social welfare structures and culture? How effective can a power, as opposed to a duty, to support private services be if those services have suffered from a long-standing under-investment in training and other resources, and can major public investment in support be justified within a market model of provision which assumes that costs should fall wholly on parents?

**The Need for a Strong Information Base**

More attention needs to be given to establishing effective information systems, at local and national levels, to underpin the development of services and strengthen the effectiveness of the Act. Our study has drawn attention on several occasions and in several areas to the inadequate information available at national and local levels.

A recent report from the EC Childcare Network, based on a review of existing data collected in Member States on services for children below compulsory school age, has discussed the potential requirements for such a system. It concludes that regular and standardised information should be collected on demand, need and use of services and on services themselves, through:

- a *survey of families* undertaken every four years; and
- an *annual 'activity report'* from each registered service, covering details of the service, children enrolled, staffing and costs and funding.

These sources of information should be collected at local authority level, to contribute to local services, then be aggregated at regional and national levels to provide a broader overview (Humblet, 1994). The emphasis therefore is on strengthening information at all levels through developing a single strategy in which the efforts of local and central government complement each other.

Examples of these methods already exist in a number of other countries. In Sweden, a national Child Care Survey is conducted annually based on a sample of 100,000 children under seven. The Survey covers users and non-users of services, and asks of both groups their preferences as well as exploring demand for services among non-users. Demographic and employment data are collected for families, but not socio-cultural characteristics, type of community or children's special needs (Möller, 1995).

Annual activity reports are also to be found in use. Since 1976, *Statistics Denmark* has collected information every year from each day care institution, plus summary information on family day care from each local authority. Information from institutions covers items about the institution itself (type, management, places, opening hours, etc.), the children attending (numbers, age distribution, payment made for the service), and staff (numbers employed full-time and part-time, total working hours per week) (Houggard, 1995). The Canadian province of Quebec collects even more detailed information on an annual basis from all day care services (Galarneau, 1995). In all three examples, the information is collected so as to be of use at a local authority as well as a national or provincial level; in Denmark, for example, statistics for local authorities are available for subscribers to the database of *Statistics Denmark*, and can be accessed by modem.

The exact content and methods for an effective information system will necessarily vary from country to country. But without effective basic management data, based on information from families and services, it is difficult to see how there can be effective monitoring of services for young children sufficient to evaluate existing policies or develop new policies for services which currently provide for over 1.5 million children and their parents.

**Looking Forward**

*Working within the existing structure*

The Children Act is now in its fifth year since implementation. It has been in operation long enough for its benefits and weaknesses to become apparent. It is a good time to take stock of the Act, at least as it applies to day care services for children under eight. This stock-taking could involve working within the existing structure of the Act and Guidance, keeping it basically intact but making amendments to improve and develop that structure in the light of experience. Within such an approach, the research team's experience points to a range of amendments that might be considered, including:

**Regulation of services:**

- the addition to the Act of a power of suspension of private day carers for whom court proceedings are pending;
- the clarification of Guidance in the following areas:
  - what constitutes 'an appropriate workload' for regulation officers;
  - the training needs and definition of core skills for officers involved in regulation;
  - the grounds on which local authorities can seek refusal/cancellation of registration;
  - compliance procedures for requirements made during annual inspections.

**Co-ordination of services**

- the extension of the section 19 Review duty to include education services, rather than as at present only requiring them to be taken into account;
- the extension of the section 19 Review duty to national government (ie. to review day care and education services regularly at a national level) or a requirement on national government to consider all local

Reviews and publish a triennial national report on early childhood services, incorporating a high level of consultation;

- the development of guidance on the sharing of information between services/agencies concerning children with disabilities, taking account of confidentiality requirements, with particular reference to day care services.

**Provision of services**

- the extension of the duty to provide for children 'in need' from day care services to day care services *and* education services for children under five;
- the extension of the duty to provide day care services for children 'in need' to a duty to provide such services *and* to ensure that providers have suitable training and support.

**Support**

- making the power to provide support into a duty, in the first place applying to providers taking children 'in need';
- the provision of guidance on what would constitute an appropriate workload for support work;
- advice to local authorities that they should ensure there is an officer with specific and exclusive responsibility for developing the support power (or duty).

More broadly, any stock-taking exercise should consider the case for and implications of extending the paramountcy principle to cover all parts of the Act, including those that apply specifically to the registration and inspection of services for children under eight. Both Guidance and Circular LAC (93)1 refer to this principle in the context of discussions about quality, standards and regulation. But these references do not mean that the principle applies legally, nor do Guidance or Circular LAC (93)1 examine the consequences were the principle to be applied to what are conceived of as private market transactions between providers and consumers (parents) in which the position and rights of the child are unclear.

*The case for a national review*

There is an argument that it is not the Act and Guidance that need review, but rather that policy on services for young children itself requires national review, to produce a set of principles and objectives that could form the basis for a national policy on services for young children, covering the full range of services (including what are currently labelled 'day care', 'education' and 'school age child care' services). As already indicated, there are a number of important but unresolved issues in services for young children that would benefit from an open, informed and thorough review process. One reason why these issues remain unresolved is that the whole field of services for young children has never been the subject of such review at national level.

There are reasons for arguing that such a review would be particularly timely at this point:

- there is an increasing need and demand for services for young children, in particular because of the rapid growth in maternal employment and a growing awareness of the importance of family support;
- at a time of increasing diversification, change and polarisation in family circumstances, it is important to take stock of the relevance and responsiveness of existing services to these circumstances;
- there have been a number of policy initiatives over the last five years in the under eights field (the implementation of the Children Act itself, the introduction and development of the childcare disregard, the Out-of-School Initiative, Home Office support for pre-school services, the voucher scheme for four year olds), which have been initiated by different departments, without a common policy framework;
- at the same time, the Children Act and now the voucher scheme both accept that 'day care' services for children over three should and can have an educational role;
- partly as the result of the success of the section 19 Review duty on local authorities, there is now a widespread recognition of the importance of regular, inclusive and well informed review as part of a process of developing policy and services and improving quality;
- there is an increasing body of knowledge, nationally and internationally, on different policy options for services for young children and their implications, and ready access to the experience and expertise of our European partners (who would also benefit from sharing British experience and expertise);

- the Government, through its adoption of the European Union Council Recommendation on Child Care in 1992 (92/241/EC), has for the first time subscribed to a set of principles and objectives for the development of services for young children.

The principles and objectives to which the Government has subscribed through adopting the Council Recommendation provide a good basis for a review of existing services and policy options since they offer criteria against which to evaluate present and future services. These principles and objectives for services include:

- accessibility (covering affordability, geographic distribution, the admission of children with special needs);
- combining reliable care with an educational approach;
- diversity and choice;
- flexibility;
- coherence between different services;
- close relations with local communities;
- responsiveness to parental needs and particular local circumstances; and
- training (both basic and continuous) for workers in services that is appropriate to the social and educative value of the work.

A review of this sort could provide not only the basis for a national policy, setting out principles, objectives and priorities, but also for a framework for the implementation of policy, covering administrative responsibility, funding, staffing, quality – and legislation. In the context of defining policy on services for young children, it would become clear whether the Children Act was the most appropriate legal basis for that policy – which might be the case if it was decided to continue with a split system model based on a distinct group of 'day care' services; or whether new legislation, for example an Early Childhood Services Act, was more suitable – which might be the case if it was decided to develop an integrated service for young children or early childhood service (for further discussion of what this alternative legislation might cover, see Moss and Penn, 1996). The Children Act has done important and useful work in carrying 'day care' services for children under eight into the 1990s, and supporting improvements; the question now is what legislative framework will best meet the needs of children and families and carry forward services for young children into the new millennium.

# References


Aldgate, J., McBeath, G., Tunstill, J., and Ozolins, R. (1994) *Implementing Section 17 of the Children Act – the first eighteen months: a study for the Department of Health,* Leicester University.

Association of Metropolitan Authorities (1991) *Children First,* London: AMA.

Audit Commission (1994) *Seen but not Heard: coordinating community child health and social services for children in need,* London: HMSO.

Audit Commission (1996) *Counting to Five: Education of Children Under Five,* London: HMSO.

Balaguer, I., Mestres, J., and Penn, H. (1991) *Quality in Services for Young Children: a discussion paper,* Brussels: European Commission Equal Opportunities Unit.

Ball, C. (1994) *Start Right: The importance of early learning,* London: Royal Society of Arts.

Ball, M. (1993) *Staff/Child Ratios in Daycare Services: an interim Report,* report to the Department of Health.

Ball, M. and Stone, J. (1991) *Setting up an Early Years Forum: a step by step guide,* London: VOLCUF.

Bond, J., Cartlidge, A., Gregson, B., Philips, P., Bolam, F., and Gill, K. (1985) *A Study of Interprofessional Collaboration in Primary Health Care Organisations,* University of Newcastle upon Tyne Health Care Research Unit.

Bone, M. (1977). *Pre-school Children and the Need for Day-Care,* London: HMSO.

Bradley, M. (1982) *The Co-ordination of Services for Children Under Five,* NFER/Nelson.

Bradshaw, J. (1990) *Child Poverty and Deprivation in the UK*, Innocenti Occasional Papers no.8, Florence: UNICEF International Child Development Centre.

Brannen, J., Mezaros, G., Moss, P. and Poland, G. (1994) *Employment and Family Life: a review of the research in the UK (1980–1994)*, London: Department of Employment Research Series no. 41.

Bull, J., Cameron, C., Candappa, M., Moss, P., Owen, C., and Statham, J. (1994a) *Implementing the Children Act for Children Under 8*, London: HMSO.

Bull, J. Cameron, C., Candappa, M., and Petrie, P. (1994b) *Provision, Regulation and Coordination of Day Care Services: a working paper from the TCRU Children Act Project*, London: Thomas Coram Research Unit, Institute of Education, University of London.

Bull, J., Cameron, C. and Moss, P. (1996) 'The 1989 Children Act: day care, welfare and early years provision', *Health and Social Care in the Community* 4 (1) 3–10.

Cameron, C. and Moss, P. (1995) 'The Children Act 1989 and early childhood services', *Journal of Social Welfare and Family Law* 17 (4) 417–429.

Cameron, C, and Statham, J. (forthcoming) 'Sponsored places: the use of sponsored day care in private and voluntary day care services', *British Journal of Social Work*.

Central Statistical Office (1995) *Social Trends 25, 1995 Edition*, London: HMSO.

Challis, L., Fuller, S., Harwood, M., Klein, R., Plowden, W., Webb, A., Whittingham, P., and Winstow, G. (1988) *Joint Approaches to Social Policy – rationality and practice*, Cambridge: CUP.

Christie, Y. and Blunden, R. (1991) *Is Race on Your Agenda?*, London: King's Fund.

Commission on Social Justice (1994) *Social Justice: Strategies for National Renewal*, London: Vintage.

DES (1990) *Starting with Quality*, Report of the Committee of Enquiry into the educational experiences offered to three and four year olds (The Rumbold Committee report), London: HMSO.

DHSS (1985) *Review of Child Care Law: Report to Ministers of an Interdepartmental Working Party*, London: HMSO.

DoH (1987) *The Law on Child Care and Family Services* (White Paper), Cmnd 62, London: HMSO.

DoH (1991) *The Children Act 1989 Guidance and Regulations (Volume 2): Family Support, Daycare and Educational Provision for Young Children*, London: HMSO.

DoH (1994) *Children Act Report 1993*, London: HMSO.

DoH (1995a) *Children's Day Care Facilities at 31 March 1992: England*, London: Department of Health.

DoH (1995b) *Moving forward: a consultation document on the regulation and inspection of social services.* London: Department of Health.

DSS (1993) *Households below Average Income: a Statistical Analysis*, London: HMSO.

Duncan, A., Giles, C., and Webb, S., (1995) *The Impact of Subsidising Childcare*, Manchester: Equal Opportunities Commission.

Dutt, R., with St. Rose, S. (undated) *Which Way Forward?* London: Race Equality Unit

EC Childcare Network (1996a) *A Review of Services for Young Children in the European Union, 1990-95*, Brussels, European Commission Equal Opportunities Unit.

EC Childcare Network (1996b) *Quality Targets in Services for Young Children*, Brussels, European Commission Equal Opportunities Unit.

Education Select Committee (House of Commons) (1989) *Educational Provision for the Under Fives, Volume II*, London: HMSO.

Elfer, P. (1993) ' Standing by standards', *Coordinate*, 35, 14.

Elfer, P. (1994). Parental views on the development of day care and education services for children under eight in England. *Early Childhood Unit Occasional Paper Series*. London: NCB.

Elfer, P. and Beasley, G. (1991) *Registration of Child minding and Day Care: Using the law to improve standards.* London: HMSO.

Elfer, P., and McQuail, S. (1996) *Local Wishes and Expectations: an evaluation of the first reviews of day care, childminding and out-of-school provision, conducted in England under Section 19 of the Children Act 1989,* London: National Children's Bureau.

Equal Opportunities Commission (1990) *The Key to Real Choice,* Manchester: Equal Opportunities Commission.

Galarneau, G. (1995) *Mise en ouevre de systèmes de collecte d'informations sur les services de garde d'enfants,* Paper given at a seminar of the EC Childcare Network on 'Reconciling employment and caring for children: what information is needed for an effective policy', Brussels, 13-14 October, 1995.

Gaster, L. and Martin, L. (1993) 'Community care planning: collaboration, co-operation and equal opportunities' *Social Services Research* no. 2, pp. 1–4 Birmingham University.

Gill, B.A.G. (1985) *Towards Genuine Consultation: principles of community participation,* Report of Joint CRE/ALAOME Conference on Multicultural Anti-racist Education, London: CRE.

Goodman A. and Wells, W. (1994) *For Richer, For Poorer: the Changing Distribution of Income in the United Kingdom 1961–1991,* London: Institute for Fiscal Studies.

Hallett, C., and Birchall, E. (1992) *Co-ordination and Child Protection,* Edinburgh: HMSO.

Harrop, A., and Moss, P. (1994) 'Working parents: trends in the 1980s' *Employment Gazette,* 102 (10) 343–352.

Hougaard, S. (1995) *Implementing systems for collecting information on childcare services: the example of Denmark,* paper given at a seminar of the EC Childcare Network on 'Reconciling employment and caring for children:

what information is needed for an effective policy', Brussels, 13-14 October, 1995.

Humblet, P. (1994) *Monitoring Childcare Services: Information Needs*, Brussels: European Commission Equal Opportunities Unit.

Hunter Johnston, E. (1996) 'Getting straight on deregulation' *Children's Services News*, January / February, 2.

Hutton, W. (1995) *The State we're in*, London: Cape.

Jenkins, S. (1994) *Winners and Losers: a Portrait of the UK Income Distribution during the 1980s (Swansea Economic Discussion Paper 94–07)*, Swansea: Department of Economics.

Kumar, V. (1993) *Poverty and Inequality in the UK: the Effects on Children*, London: National Children's Bureau.

Littlewood, J. (1994) *Evaluation: the role of social research*, London: HMSO.

Marsh, A. and McKay, S. (1993). 'Families, work and the use of childcare' *Employment Gazette*, August, 361–370.

McQuail, S. and Pugh. G. (1995) *Effective Organisation of Early Childhood*, London: National Children's Bureau.

McRae, S. (1991) *Maternity rights in Britain: the PSI Report on the Experience of Women and Employers*, London: Policy Studies Institute.

Meltzer, H. (1994). *Day Care Services For Children*. London: HMSO..

Möller, E. (1995) *Information collected in Sweden on leave and childcare services*, paper given at a seminar of the EC Childcare Network on 'Reconciling employment and caring for children: what information is needed for an effective policy', Brussels, 13–14 October, 1995.

Moss, P. (1992) 'Employee child care', *Employee Relations*, 14 (6) 20–32.

Moss, P., and Owen, C. (1989) 'Use of pre-school day care and education 1979–86', *Children and Society*, 3 (4) 296–310.

Moss, P. and Penn, H. (1996) *Transforming Nursery Education,* London: Paul Chapman Publishing.

Moss, P., Owen, C., Statham, J., Bull, J., Cameron, C., and Candappa, M. (1995) *Survey of Day Care Providers in England and Wales: a working paper from the TCRU Children Act project*. London: Thomas Coram Research Unit, Institute of Education, University of London.

Mulford, C., and Rogers, D. (1982) 'Definitions and models' in (ed.) Rogers, D. and Whetten, D. A., and Associates, *Interorganisational Coordination: theory, research and implementation,* Iowa: Iowa State University Press.

National Commission on Education (1993) *Learning to Succeed: a radical look at education today and a strategy for the future,* London: Heinemann.

National Consumer Council (1991) *Daycare Services for Under Fives: the consumer view,* NCC.

NPDNA (1993) *Report of the Survey of Members' Experiences of Re-registration Under the Children Act 1989,* Nottingham: NES Arnold.

Office of Population Censuses and Surveys (OPCS)(1995) *General Household Survey 1993,* London: HMSO.

Owen, C., and Moss, P. (1989) 'Patterns of pre-school provision in English local authorities', *Journal of Educational Policy,* 4, 309–28.

Penn, H., and Riley, K. (1992) *Managing Services for the Under Fives*. Essex: Longman.

Pugh, G. (1992a) An Equal Start for all our Children? TRS/Greenwich Lecture.

Pugh, G. (1992b) *Contemporary Issues in the Early Years,* London: Paul Chapman.

Qaiyoom, R. (1992) *From Crisis to Consensus: a strategic approach for local government and the black voluntary sector,* London: SIA.

Schweinhart, L. J., and Weikart, D. P. (1993) *A Summary of Significant Benefits: the High Scope Perry Preschool Study Through age 27*, Michigan: High Scope UK.

Shephard, G (1995) *Oral Statement by the Secretary of State for Education*, 6 July.

Sherriff, C. (1995) 'Transatlantic child care', *Child Care Now*, 15 (1 and 2) 17.

Smith, T., (1990) 'Services for the Under Fives – what children need and parents want?', *Local Government Policy Making*, 17 (3) 56–60.

SSI (1994) *Telling the Day Care Story*, London: DoH.

Statham, J. (1993) *The Children Act and Under Eights in Wales*, London: Thomas Coram Research Unit, Institute of Education, University of London.

Statham, J. (1996) *Young Children in Wales: an evaluation of the implementation of the Children Act 1989 for day care services*, London: Thomas Coram Research Unit, Institute of Education, University of London.

Statham, J., and Cameron, C. (1994) 'Young children in rural areas: implementing the Children Act', *Children and Society*, 8 (1) 17–30.

Statham, J., Lloyd, E., Moss, P., Melhuish, E., and Owen, C. (1990) *Playgroups in a Changing World*, London: HMSO.

VOLCUF (undated) Why have an Early Years Forum?/Checklist for an Effective Forum (mimeo) London: VOLCUF.

Whetten, D.A. (1981) Interorganisational relations: a review of the field, *Journal of Higher Education*, 52 (1) 1–28.

APPENDIX
1

# Publications from the Children Act Studies in England and Wales

**conducted by the Thomas Coram Research Unit, Institute of Education University of London**

**Books, Reports and Working Papers**

Bull, J., Cameron, C., Candappa, M., Moss, P., Owen, C. and Statham, J. (1994) *Implementing the Children Act for Children under 8*, London: HMSO.

Bull, J., Cameron, C., Candappa, M. and Petrie, P. (1994) *Provision, Regulation and Coordination of Day Care Services (TCRU Children Act Project Working Paper No. 1)*, London: Thomas Coram Research Unit, Institute of Education, University of London.

Moss, P., Owen, C., Statham, J., Bull, J., Cameron, C. and Candappa, M. (1995) *Survey of Day Care providers in England and Wales (TCRU Children Act Project Working Paper No. 2)*, London:, Thomas Coram Research Unit, Institute of Education, University of London.

Statham, J. (1993) *The Children Act and Under 8s in Wales*, London: Thomas Coram Research Unit, Institute of Education, University of London.

Statham, J. (1996) *Young Children in Wales: an evaluation of the implementation of the Children Act 1989 for day care services*, London: Thomas Coram Research Unit, Institute of Education, University of London.

**Academic Journals and Book Chapters**

Bull, J. (1996) 'Implementing the Children Act: the regulation of day care services for young children', *British Journal of Social Work*, 26, 53–75.

Bull, J., Cameron, C. and Moss, P. (1996) 'The 1989 Children Act: welfare, day care and early years provision', *Health and Social Care in the Community*, 4(1), 3–10.

Cameron, C. and Moss, P. (1995) 'The Children Act 1989 and early childhood services', *Journal of Social Welfare and Family Law*, 17(4), 433–466.

Cameron, C. and Statham, J. (forthcoming) 'Sponsored places: the use of independent day care services to support children in need', *British Journal of Social Work.*

Candappa, M. (1994) ' Equal opportunities and ethnicity in the early years: implementing the Children Act', *Children & Society,* 8 (3), 218–231.

Statham, J. (1996, forthcoming) 'Local planning of services for young children: the role of the Section 19 day care reviews in Wales', in Cohen, B. and Hagen, U. (eds) *Children's Services: shaping up for the millennium,* Edinburgh: HMSO.

Statham, J. and Cameron, C. (1994) 'Young children in rural areas: implementing the Children Act', *Children & Society,* 8(1), 17–30.

**Other Publications**

Cameron, C. (1994) 'Services for under eights', *Children Act News,* 14, 5.

Candappa, M. (1995) 'Equal opportunities and ethnicity in early childhood services', *Childcare Now,* 15(3), 10–11.

Candappa, M. (1996) 'Under 8s services and the Children Act', *Children's Services News.*

Candappa, M. (1996) 'Working together in services for young children', *Coordinate.*

Statham, J. (1995) *Archwiliad o ofalwyr dydd yng Nghymru (summary of a survey of day care providers in Wales),* London: Thomas Coram Research Unit, Institute of Education, University of London.

Statham, J. (1996) 'Family planning', *Community Care,* 1101, 28–29.